PRAISE FOR FORK IN THE ROAD

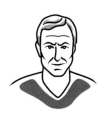

"Medical professionals now agree that nothing is more harmful in our diets than the refined carbs and sugars we consume. Even so, many of us still struggle to change the way we eat and, by doing so, improve both our mental and physical health. Carbohydrate addiction might be the key. Fork in the Road is the simple, beautiful book that explains how to do this. Dr Jen Unwin has given us the ideal guide to freeing yourself from the fattening carbs in the diet and finally getting healthy."

GARY TAUBES, Author of **THE CASE FOR KETO** and **WHY WE GET FAT**

"Sugar isn't tobacco, alcohol, or heroin. It's worse. Because we give it to children and call it love. The keys to cutting sugar and increasing love are within these pages."

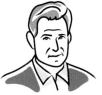

ROBERT LUSTIG, MD, MSL
Author of **FAT CHANCE** and **METABOLICAL**

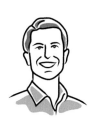

High sugar and refined carbohydrate diets have been shown to contribute to many serious long-term health problems including type 2 diabetes and heart disease. If you want better health, wellbeing and immunity, a diet free of these foods is key. Every day I speak to people struggling to break free and eat well. Fork in the Road can start you on your journey to a healthier and happier life today.

ASEEM MALHORTA, MD, MSL
Author of **THE PIOPPI DIET** and **THE 21-DAY IMMUNITY PLAN**

As with any adjustment to your diet or exercise regimen, consult your doctor before implementing changes. If you have a medical issue that you are concerned about, consult your health care practitioner. The authors and publishers will not be liable for any complications, injuries, loss, or other medical problem arising from or in connection with using this book.

Copyright © 2021 by Jen Unwin, Psy D, FBPSs, C Psychol

All rights reserved. No portion of this book may be reproduced — mechanically, electronically, or by any other mans, including photocopying-without written permission of the publisher.

ISBN 9798714538025
1. Health 2. Self-care 3. Nutrition

Dr Jen Unwin is a clinical psychologist. And a lifelong carbohydrate addict. Fork in the Road guides you in a clear way to identifying if you have carbohydrate addiction, finding the motivation to change your life, understanding how to build the right daily eating plan, the strategies for long-term success, and where to go for more information and support.
In this beautifully illustrated book, Jen teams up with top clinicians in the field and with creative low-carbers who share what they have learned about freeing yourself from the emotional and physical dangers of overeating sugars, flours and processed foods. Make today your 'Fork in the Road' to health and food freedom.

Published by FITR Publishing
ForkInTheRoad.co.uk

Version 2021.08.12
August 2021

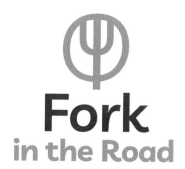

Fork
in the Road

*A Hopeful Guide to
Food Freedom*

DR JEN UNWIN

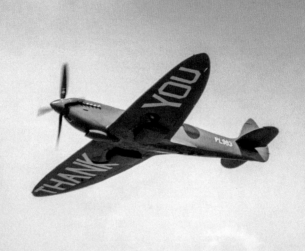

Everyone we meet shapes us. If we are lucky, we might encounter a few true soul mates on our journey. Many of the thoughts and ideas in this book have developed out of conversations with my remarkable husband, David.

I met my best friend, Kate at the age of 8. It was a sweet time in every way! Now we spend our pocket money on knitting supplies not pear drops.

My Mum once said to me that I had brought her up and I feel the same about you, Katie, Rob, and Edward.

Special thanks to Georgia Ede, Anna Fruehling, Bitten Jonsson, and Dave Wolfe for sharing their expertise on food, the brain, and addiction. Kiki Johnson, Micheal Rowley, and Katie Caldesi have very special creativity and it's been a honour to work with them on this project.

The author's profits from the sales of this book go to

Public Health Collaboration PHCuk.org.

A charity close to my heart that campaigns

for better public health information.

YOUR FORK IN THE ROAD CREW

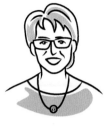

@Jen_Unwin

Dr Jen Unwin, Clinical Psychologist
ForkInTheRoad.co.uk

Jen worked for 32 years in the NHS helping people with chronic health problems to improve their quality of life. She gained her doctorate in the importance of hope in healthcare outcomes. She now combines this knowledge with her own experience of carb addiction to support Dr Unwin helping patients to give up sugar and carbohydrates to improve their health.

I've pulled together a crack team of experts on carbohydrate addiction and glued them together with Kiki and Michael's creativity and my own knowledge and experience. This is the book I wish I had found four decades ago. I know that the knowledge here will help you take a different path. The path to food freedom and sugar sobriety. Please let me know how you get on via Twitter @Jen_Unwin or via the website ForkInTheRoad.co.uk

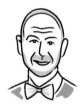

@LowCarbGP

Dr David Unwin , GP

David has been helping patients in his practice to reverse type 2 diabetes and other health conditions by advising a low carb diet. He has written a number of academic papers on the results and spoken internationally. David was named NHS Innovator of the year for his work in 2016. He has appeared on TV and his work has been covered by The Times and The New Scientist.

I believe we have eaten our way into the triple pandemics of obesity, diabetes and fatty liver disease. I also believe we can eat our way out by eating tasty real food. Every day my patients achieve this miracle and you can too.

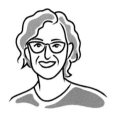

Dr Georgia Ede
DiagnosisDiet.com

Georgia is a Harvard-trained psychiatrist who believes that what we eat is the biggest factor in our mental and physical health. She suffered from a range of mystery complaints in her 40's which she eventually cured by following a very low carbohydrate and high fat diet. She has been incorporating nutrition into her practice for over a decade and is passionate about sharing her knowledge of the brain and nutrition to benefit others. She lectures widely and has appeared on many podcasts.

@GeorgiaEdeMD

No amount of the food(s) you are addicted to will satisfy you. Chasing that feeling is a hollow, delusional, and demoralizing pursuit. As hard as it sometimes is to resist the first bite, it is infinitely harder...and usually virtually impossible...to resist the second...and the third...and the fourth. If you give in to that first bite, all the insight, motivation, hard work, and experience in the world won't usually be enough to prevent full relapse.

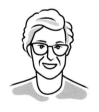

Anna Fruehling
SUGARxGlobal.com

Anna is a certified primal health coach and is 31 years in recovery from drugs and alcohol. She only recognised she was a sugar junkie after she heard Bitten Jonsson speaking at an online summit. She is now committed to helping people with sugar addiction and works closely with Dave Wolfe. Her passion and enthusiasm are infectious. She runs the Facebook group Peace of Keto.

@FruehlingAnna

One day is a day won! You deserve to feel energetic, interesting, and whole. The freedom you get from quitting sugar and learning how to live without addiction is more than you can imagine. You are giving up something that is harming you, not something good. You are GAINING so much more.

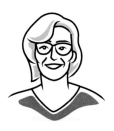

@BittenJonsson

Bitten Jonsson

BittensAddiction.com

Bitten is an internationally renowned expert on sugar addiction. She is a registered nurse and has been helping sugar addicts for decades. She now teaches others to assess and treat sugar addiction. She first understood addiction during her treatment for alcohol use in the USA and then came to see that sugar was a gateway drug. She is a much-respected pioneer in this field.

I wish a book like this had been available when I started out, I was seen as crazy here in Sweden, not eating "normally". The most common question I have had over the years is 'When are you going to be "normal"?' My answer is with a laugh, 'But you know I am normal'. I also like to point out that without other like-minded fellow travelers on this journey I do not think I would have made it. Group support is incredibly important and so is knowledge about neuroscience and the addicted brain, that's power.

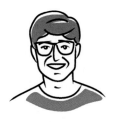

@TriggerFree_RD

Dave Wolfe

TriggerFreeNutrition.com

David is a registered dietitian, food addiction counsellor and sugar addiction coach. He learned about food addiction from his mother, Judy Wolfe and soon realised that he too suffered from it. He has trained with some of the most knowledgeable people worldwide, including Bitten. He is passionate about the recovery community and offers free weekly meetings.

No one is beyond hope! I've seen miracles take place every day, you can recover and you can learn a new way to live.

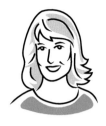

Katie Caldesi

LowCarbTogether.com

Katie is a cook and food writer. With her chef husband Giancarlo she has two restaurants and a cookery school. When Giancarlo was diagnosed with coeliac disease and type 2 diabetes they had to learn a new way of eating and cooking. Katie is passionate about sharing her knowledge and has written a number of beautiful low carb cook books.

@KatieCaldesi

My husband Giancarlo is a self-confessed sugar addict but with a combined effort from the whole family we have removed temptations from our kitchen and replaced them with delicious healthy foods for him to enjoy instead. Treats still appear but they are no longer bars of milk chocolate, biscuits or raisins that harmed him so much. He has been in remission from type 2 diabetes for 8 years now.

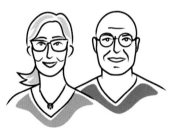

Kiki Johnson & Michael Rowley

CreativeKi.com

Kiki and Michael are a wife and husband team who run a design and branding studio. Their shift to focusing on health and wellness clients was inspired by Michael's health recovery brought about by fasting, meditation, and especially Kiki's delicious, low-carb meals.

@CreateKi

Michael: I turned to a low-carb way of eating after a physical showed I was on my way to having the same ailments that killed my father: obesity and diabetes — and ultimately pancreatic cancer and dementia. Saddened by my father's death, my mother turned to high-carb comfort foods. With the onset of dementia, she was having frequent foggy days. With gentle nudging she switched to a low-carb diet, lost 45 pounds (20kg), and went from having difficulty walking to dancing with joy. Switching to keto meals, her mental clarity and healthspan greatly improved.

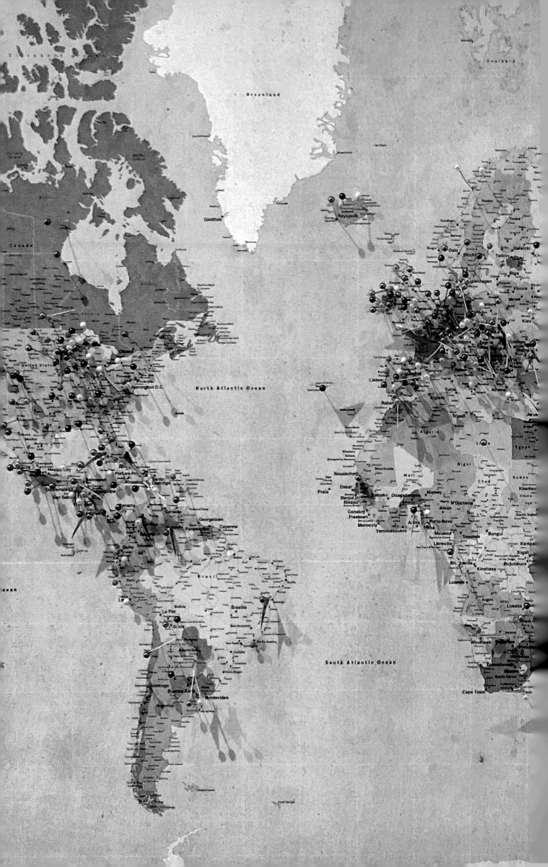

Forward

I am Dr David Unwin, a GP in Northern England from 1986. Since starting work as a young doctor I have seen a growing epidemic of obesity and diabetes.

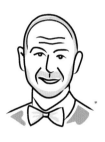

DAVID

In the early days, people with significant weight problems were quite rare. Now every clinic brings people suffering the painful consequences of eating too much; back and knee pain, high blood pressure, Type 2 Diabetes, fatty liver disease, and mental illnesses like depression. Some patients have all of these. For years I prescribed different drugs for each of these conditions but began to realize each drug was just a 'sticking plaster' which didn't address the basic problem, which was what my patients were eating. Even worse, some of the drugs were giving side effects that needed yet more drugs to counteract them!

In the US more than half of all adults 65 and older (54%) report taking four or more prescription drugs. In my clinical experience many of these people on multiple medications don't actually feel well. Around 2012 I started looking for the actual causes of these problems, particularly Type 2 Diabetes. This led me to the low carbohydrate diet and for the first time to working clinically with my wife, Jen. I needed her help as a clinical health psychologist because of her expertise around behaviour change. I had come to realise that the answers to so many chronic illnesses lie in not drugs but in lifestyle change. Who are the experts in this? Psychologists! I was married to one who would help me for free. Bingo! Jen's doctorate was on the role of hope in chronic disease and as we worked together, I came to see first-hand how powerful hope was in changing behaviour.

Before, I tended to just tell patients what to do, whereas Jen taught me to factor in personal goals and supply feedback. (As you will learn in Chapter 2.) This helped revolutionise medicine for me, for the first time I was collaborating with my patients, working towards shared goals. Such cheerful, happy medicine! Partly as a result of this, the practice started spending less on drugs. We now spend £50,000 ($68,000) less per year on drugs for diabetes than is average for our area. This was humbling for me as I came to see how fundamental psychology was to good medicine.

As we worked with people cutting sugar and starchy foods from their diet, Jen and I were struck by how much happier they seemed. Some even came off antidepressants after many years. Again and again we saw how a better diet seemed to change peoples' whole attitude to life. Indeed, when Jen and I went low-carb alongside our patients I became more confident, less anxious and needed a lot less sleep. We were experiencing how diet could change our brains and mental attitude. You will learn more about how this occurs in Chapter 5.

Jen and I have known each other since childhood. (Our mothers were best friends.) I can testify that her weight went up and down all that time, by about three stone (20kg/44 pounds). She seemed to go through cycles that required whole wardrobes with clothes of different sizes.

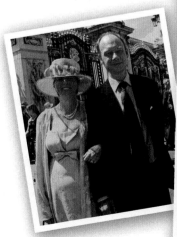

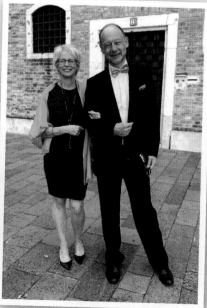

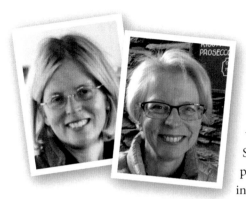

This was a typical cycle: Jen would tell me she hated being so overweight and she had found yet another new diet to try. In the lead up to 'the diet' she seemed to panic and eat more, and more! Suddenly there were tray bakes and puddings. Then the new diet would start in earnest. I liked this phase because Jen was happier and felt in control again. She always lost lots of weight and soon looked and felt fabulous, but I would become anxious for her as I knew it would not last. The end could be Christmas, a holiday or just a meal out. I noticed her eating change but learnt that criticism didn't help. I wasn't telling her anything she didn't already know after all. Very soon all the weight would be back.

Meanwhile in our low carb work there were patients who seemed to struggle in a similar way to Jen. **They would initially do well, then Christmas or a birthday came and all the weight would pile back on.** Jen and I had a slow, painful, dawning realization that these people and herself had some similarities with other groups I knew well; smokers and people struggling with alcohol. After many decades here was a model that fitted so well; sugar and other carbohydrate foods as an addiction. Just as with alcohol the remedy was simple but really not easy; abstinence. In Chapters 1 and 6 you can read more about how Jen helped herself and many of my patients.

I have discussed the idea of food addiction with people I have looked after for 30 years who have cried with relief to discover they are not mad or alone after all. Having never told anyone about their abnormal relationship with bread or cornflakes, they finally have a model to help them understand their behaviour. It took Jen a few years to eliminate all her trigger foods. (There were a lot!) This has involved sacrifices I never thought she could achieve (like alcohol, nuts and cheese), but the benefits to Jen's self-esteem and peace of mind are worth it. I have seen similar transformations in some of our patients. One young person recently presented with sleep apnoea, requesting bariatric surgery to put an end to it all. A year later, off carbs and sugar, off booze and off cigarettes they are eight stone down (51 kilos/112 pounds) and have started jogging!

Carbohydrates, sugars and sources of glucose explained

There are some areas of nutrition where it is easy to become confused. For example what are 'carbs' and when we talk of 'sugar' do we mean the stuff we buy in bags, or glucose? The foods we eat are composed of proteins, fats and carbohydrates; what nutritionists call the three macronutrients.

The Three Macronutrients

PROTEIN   FAT   CARBS

Carbohydrates, as the name suggests, are made of three elements; carbon, hydrogen and oxygen. Plants manufacture them to store energy from the sun using the process of photosynthesis, where carbon dioxide is combined with water. The simplest sugars are also known as monosaccharides, which literally means "one sugar". Glucose is among the most important of these and the one people with diabetes struggle to metabolise. Another common monosaccharide is fructose found in fruits and honey (more on this later). If you combine glucose and fructose you have a disaccharide, a mixture of two sugars, in this case called sucrose, the sugar we use to sweeten our tea.

Note, the proper names of sugars end in -ose, and there are lots of others like maltose (in beer), lactose (in milk) and dextrose. But back to sucrose, the equal mix of fructose and glucose, in common parlance this is just called 'sugar' but to save confusion in this book we will call sucrose 'table sugar'.

Fructose
Sugar from Fruit & Honey

Glucose
Simple Sugar from Plants

Sucrose
Fructose + Glucose (Table Sugar)

Lactose
Sugar from Milk

Maltose
Sugar in Beer

Dextrose
Sugar from Corn

If you make a huge 'supermolecule' by joining lots of glucose molecules together you just made starch. This is the way plants have found to store lots of these sugars. The process of digestion breaks starchy foods like bread, rice, potatoes or breakfast cereals back down into surprising quantities of glucose.

Starch Molecule

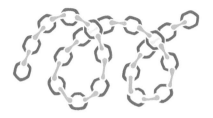

Glucose molecules are bonded together in long spiraling starch molecules

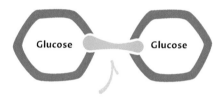

Glycosidic Bond

Digestion breaks the bonds
Bread tastes sweet when you chew it as saliva enzymes break glycosidic bonds

Some of you will have heard of the 'Low GI' diet. This refers to the Glycaemic Index which ranks carbohydrates in terms of how much they put up blood sugar (or more properly blood glucose) relative to pure glucose, which counts as 100. We used the same glycaemic index and the related glycaemic load to produce infographics to help people understand how foods might affect their blood glucose compared to a teaspoon of table sugar. For example, a small bowl of rice (150 grams) will put your blood glucose up to approximately the same extent as ten teaspoons of table sugar. This is why if you are overweight, have diabetes or pre-diabetes it can make sense to avoid not just table sugar but starchy carbs, replacing them with green vegetables, meat, fish, dairy and nuts. This is the basis of the low carb diet and also the delicious recipes you will find in Chapter 4.

Our diets contain three common sources of sugar-rich foods
- Naturally sweet foods like honey, raisins, apples or bananas.
- Foods sweetened with table sugar like cakes, biscuits or many 'low fat' foods.
- Starchy carbohydrates that digest down into glucose like bread, potatoes, or rice.

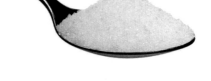

Our Sugar Burden
Three Sources of Sugar Consumption
4-Gram Teaspoon of Table Sugar Equivalents Per 100 grams/mls*

Naturally Occurring Sugars	Foods with Added Sugars	Food Digested Into Sugars
Banana	**Chocolate Rice Crispies**	**Brown Bread**
4.9 tsp	**24.4 tsp**	**10.8 tsp**
Honey	**Fizzy Orange** (1/3 CAN)	**Boiled Spaghetti**
17.6 tsp	**1.0 tsp**/100ml	**3.7 tsp**
Skimmed Milk	**Digestive Biscuits**	**French Fries**
0.9 tsp	**8.8 tsp**	**5.1 tsp**
Raisins	**Malt Loaf**	**Basmati Rice**
17.1 tsp	**14.7 tsp**	**6.8 tsp**
Apple Juice	**Raspberry Yoghurt**	**Baked Potato**
4.3 tsp	**2.4 tsp**	**6.3 tsp**

*As each food would effect blood glucose, from the International tables of glycaemic index and glycaemic load (Atkinson, Foster-Powell et at. 2008) as per the calculations in a paper published in The Journal of Insulin Resistance "It's The Glycaemic Response To, Not The Carbohydrate Content of Food That Matters in Diabetes and Obesity: The Glycaemic Index Revisited.' D J Unwin et al.

Many people are astonished to learn a 200 ml (7 ounce) glass of pure apple juice has approximately the same effect on blood glucose as eight teaspoons of table sugar or that 100 grams (about three slices) of brown bread is equivalent to more than ten teaspoons.

The observant amongst you may have noticed that by comparing foods to a teaspoon of table sugar (the disaccharide sucrose) instead of pure glucose we have added another variable; fructose. We did this because my patients struggled to understand glucose as a substance (they were unfamiliar with it) and the glycaemic load gives a result in grams (they used ounces). I wanted a comparator that was familiar (the standard 4 gram teaspoon of table sugar).

Although fructose (fruit sugar) is sweeter than table sugar it does not put blood glucose up directly. For a while this led to the belief it was a safe food. However, we now know it is not an innocent bystander. Professor Robert Lustig, Professor of Paediatric Endocrinology at the University of California, has devoted much of his professional life to helping the world see the perils of fructose, especially the fructose in the high fructose corn syrup added to so many foods and drinks. As Professor Lustig points out, fructose puts a particular strain on the liver, in a very similar way to alcohol.

I have come to understand there are as many individual diets as there are people. Jen and I are on a low carb diet but in reality, Jen's low carb diet is not the same as mine. It can be a long journey to find a diet that suits you and achieves your goals. Personal preferences, food intolerances, socioeconomic factors, religion, ethical beliefs, ability/motivation to cook and many other factors affect your choices. However, with respect to choice, for many of us there is a snag. You may well choose to eat chocolate bars or Doritos and on discovering the health consequences try to cut back, only to be surprised by cravings and find yourself unable to stop. For some of us the crocodile in the waters of choice is food addiction. If this is you, this little book is here to help. Jen has written it in the hope that some of you can be helped without having to wait thirty years like she did.

*Start your journey
to more control, better health,
and improved wellbeing*

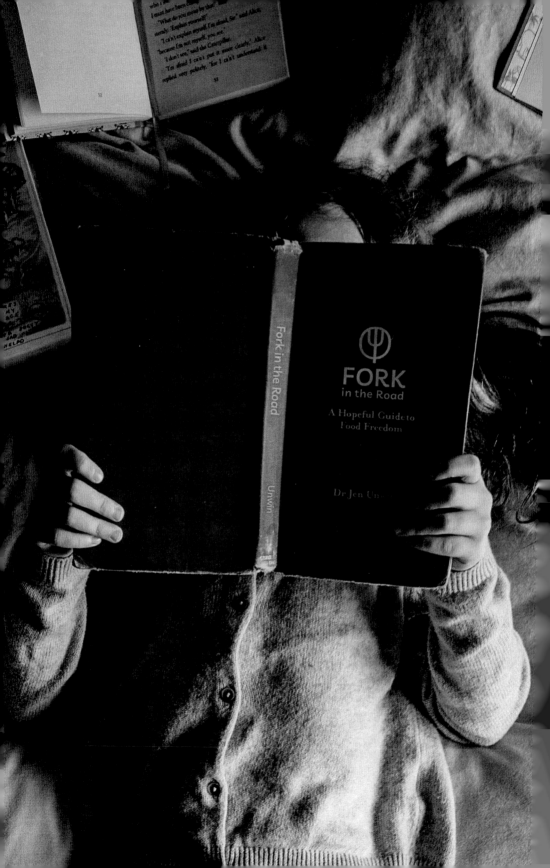

Introduction

*I have tried to write the book I wish
I had stumbled upon 46 years ago.
If only I had this knowledge at the age of 10
it would have saved A LOT of heartache.*

*My aim is to share with you what I now know about
sugar addiction and how to escape its grip.*

This knowledge has finally enabled me to overcome decades of struggles with weight, food cravings and the growing hopelessness of finding a long-term solution. I want to spread a little light to those of you still trying to find your own path forward to food freedom. I have sprinkled each chapter with advice and wisdom from fellow sugar addicts and experts in the field. If this book helps you, I sincerely hope you will also in turn reach out to help others.

My brightest early memory is of some warm cheese scones, covered in melting butter. I was maybe 4 years old. I already loved sugar and carbohydrate heavy foods. I saved all my pocket money to spend on sweets. Food was front and centre in our family and I'm pretty sure looking back my Mum was a fellow addict. The tragic death of my father's brother and then his own life-threatening illness put a strain on the family when I was still only young and I turned increasingly to food for comfort and amusement. I loved sneaking food from the kitchen; buttered toast, hot milk with loads of sugar, condensed milk, baking chocolate or whatever was available. I also adored baking and cooking, so was an avid maker of cakes, biscuits and puddings. Needless to say, by 12 years old I was over 12 stone (170 lb) or 76 kilos in new money. I hated being overweight but looking back can see I was already addicted to sugar. I got the shakes if I couldn't eat regularly and eating was how I managed boredom and other emotional states.

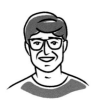 **DAVID** *I remember getting home from kindergarten, running downstairs and grabbing 5 pouches of fruit snacks, eating them in a handful and hiding the wrappers.*

GEORGIA *When my sisters and I were young, my mom would give us each a dollar on the first of every month to buy whatever we wanted or save up for something special. I always chose sour cream and onion potato chips and a bag of M&Ms. When I was about 10 years old I remember sneaking down into the kitchen after dark to get a banana. I went back to bed and ate it under my covers so my mom wouldn't catch me. People say fruit isn't sugar...but my cravings for fruit were just as strong as my cravings for chips, candy, and ice cream. The only thing I've ever stolen in my whole life was a Choco'Lite candy bar. We didn't have much money so I couldn't ask my mom to buy one for me. It was brand new on the market so my favorite TV shows were littered with commercials showing winged Choco-Lite bars flying through the air. I couldn't stop thinking about trying one. I was about 8 years old.*

I went on several crazy diets with my mum over my young teenage years. Egg and grapefruit was a memorable one. I finally managed to lose 20 kilograms when I was 16 and absolutely determined to get a boyfriend! The magic formula was boiled eggs for breakfast, apple and Edam cheese for lunch and dinner without the carby part of the meal or pudding. I was thrilled with what I'd achieved but hadn't yet understood that I would never be able to moderate my relationship with sugar and carbohydrate. So, when it crept back into my diet, the weight crept back on. This ushered in decades of dieting, followed by weight re-gain and a cycle of misery. Meanwhile, I succeeded in all other areas of my life. I qualified as a Clinical Psychologist and had a career I loved. I married my wonderful husband and we made a beautiful family. Still, I struggled with food cravings, weight gain and increasingly desperate attempts to maintain a healthy weight. I really disliked being overweight but I really loved eating, it seemed like an unsolvable puzzle.

GEORGIA *When I was about 13 years old, I remember crying to my mom about how hard it was to lose weight, and how unfair it seemed that most of the other kids in my class seemed to effortlessly maintain a normal weight without having to count calories, exercise, or feel hungry all the time.*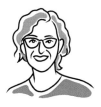

Finally, at 48 years old I stumbled across a book by Dr John Briffa called "Escape the Diet Trap' in the sale section at the supermarket. This was to be my 'fork in the road' moment and the beginning of my food freedom journey. The knowledge in the book was about low carbohydrate or keto diets and why they work. I understood the science and dove straight in, going cold turkey from sugar and carbohydrates. I felt pretty grim for about 8 days whilst my body learned to burn fat instead of glucose for fuel but soon felt better than I had for years both mentally and physically. My husband, David and I later took this knowledge and started to help patients at his GP practice to reverse their diabetes and other chronic health conditions. We were both amazed at the results people were able to achieve and have written 8 academic papers and even appeared on the BBC 'The Truth about Carbs' program which had 4 million viewers. Four hundred and sixty thousand people have now done the online low carb program we helped design. We've been privileged to speak all over the world.

Low carb eating was a big part of the answer for me and many others but not the whole story. It was the start. Lots of things have tripped me up along the way and sent me back into weight gain and struggles with food cravings. There was much more for me to learn personally about staying in recovery from sugar and carbohydrate addiction. The information that has been most useful to me about food but also about understanding addiction is in the following chapters. I am not smug. I have no doubt I will have future struggles with food but I now have the knowledge and support to regain the right path and that is what I'll share with you.

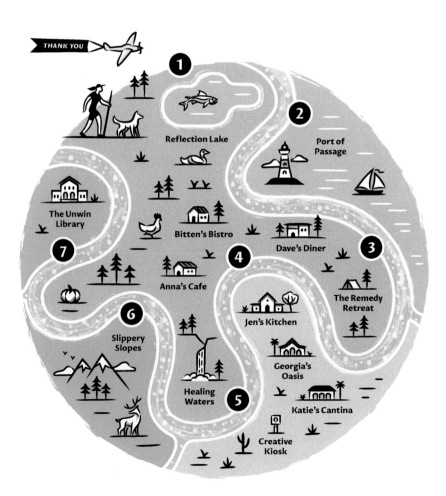

A Hopeful Guide to Food Freedom

Chapter 1 : Are You a Carbohydrate Addict?   25
The nature of carbohydrate addiction. We'll help you to identify if you most likely are experiencing it. I'll also explain the ways in which certain foods can be addictive.

Chapter 2 : Your Passport to Recovery   37
Planning your recovery journey and how to stick the course. Like any important journey or project there will be struggles and setbacks, so finding your motivation and can-do is priority number one.

Chapter 3 : The Problem and The Remedy   45
What should I eat and not eat?

Chapter 4 : Recipes   61
Food addiction recovery is not about deprivation, so we'll explore all the wonderful things you can eat. We'll set out some sample meal plans and delicious, easy recipes to get you going. You can make the advice work for you and make it fit your own life and goals. There is no one solution that fits everyone.

Chapter 5 : Healing Your Addicted Brain   109
Once you've got into eating like a recovered sugar addict, then we will delve deeper into how sugar affects the brain and how to heal for long-term success.

Chapter 6 : Slips, Trips, and Falls   123
Lapses are part of the recovery journey. It's how you handle them that's important.

Chapter 7 : Resources   141
A detailed list of resources to help you into the future with even more knowledge: podcasts, support groups, websites and books.

Let's step out together on your carb addiction recovery journey!
I hope some of you will remember this book as your 'fork in the road'
in years to come.

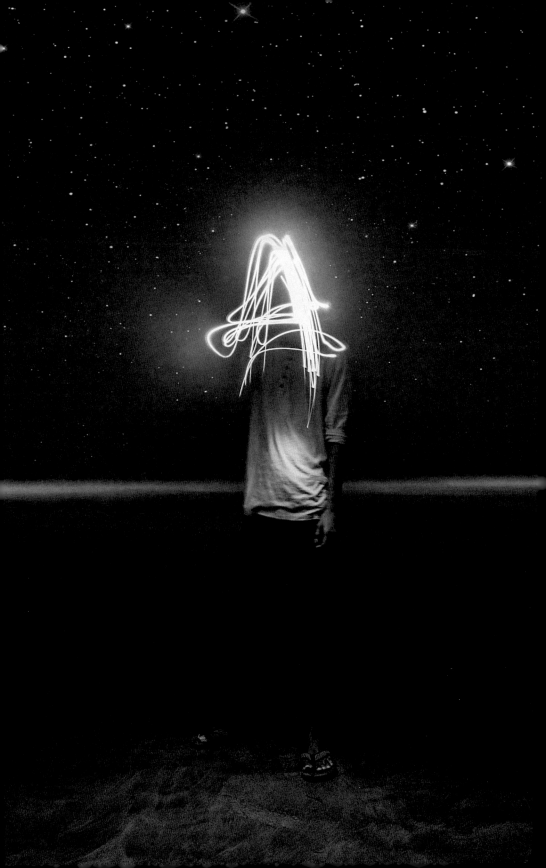

CHAPTER 1

Are You a Carbohydrate Addict?

*Once I had heard the idea of sugar addiction,
I immediately recognised myself and was able
to use this new perspective to understand
and improve my relationship
with food and my body.*

BITTEN *I learned I was addicted to alcohol when
I was thrown in to a treatment center in California
in 1985, that's the best thing that ever happening to
me, although I was devastated at first. But when I
learned addiction is a brain illness and I learned
about all the neuroscience. Being a nurse, I fell in
love with addiction medicine and have been devoted to it ever since.*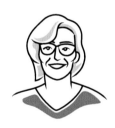

*After seven years being sober, I found myself hiding, lying and sneaking with
chocolate and ice cream and deep inside I understood, I am a sugar addict,
and was one long before alcohol came in to my life. In fact, sugar sensitized
my reward center so alcohol hit harder. Once I admitted that, my recovery
began and my life totally turned around. For me understanding and having
knowledge is the power that drives my recovery. The information in this
chapter is vital for all sugar and carb addicts.*

Although there is doubt and debate amongst some researchers and clinicians as to whether sugar addiction is 'real', there are plenty of us who now embrace it as explaining our struggles.

Once I had heard the idea of carb addiction, I immediately recognised myself and was able to use this new perspective to understand and improve my relationship with food and my body. I couldn't believe that as a clinical psychologist I hadn't recognised it earlier. I'm sure if we were to survey the general public then a high proportion would agree that certain foods can be addictive.

GEORGIA
A client recently told me
"I could do a face plant in
a bowl of rice."

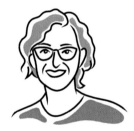

Some people call it food addiction and some sugar addiction. Here I will mostly use the term 'carbohydrate' addiction which covers all sugars and starches. As Dr Unwin explained in the introduction, starches are made up of glucose molecules. This is why starchy foods can have a considerable amount of 'sugar' in them. In fact, the starch molecule is made up of joined up glucose molecules which explains how a 150-gram bowl of boiled rice may affect your blood sugar by as much as 10 teaspoons of table sugar.

Most carbohydrate addicts struggle with foods containing both sugar and carbohydrate, often in combination with fat. In my experience pure fats and proteins are not problematic. Think about how often you have met anyone who had out of control cravings for steak or lard! More on food in Chapter 3.

But what is addiction?

The American Society of Addiction Medicine defines addiction as follows:

'Addiction is a treatable, chronic medical disease involving complex interactions among brain circuits, genetics, the environment, and an individual's life experiences. People with addiction use substances or engage in behaviors that become compulsive and often continue despite harmful consequences.'

In my opinion, this applies to food consumption for some people. Many of us certainly have an ongoing struggle with moderating certain foods despite experiencing harmful physical and mental consequences. The message of hope is that this addiction is treatable as you will see in this book.

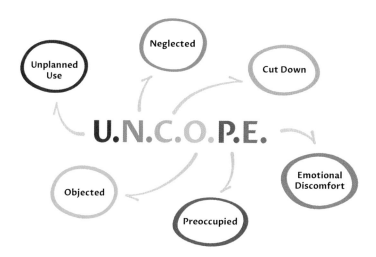

UNCOPE is an easy way to 'screen' yourself

Take this quick questionnaire developed by our wonderful expert, Bitten Jonsson based on the World Health Organisation criteria.

UNCOPE Screening

Sweets* can be any carbohydrate such as pasta, bread, desserts, biscuits, fizzy drinks, ice cream, pizza, cereal, potatoes, rice, sweeteners, with or without fat etc.

Yes   **No**

○   ○   **1. U = Unplanned use**
In the past year, have you ever eaten more sweets* than you intended or have you spent more time eating, using sweets* than you intended to?"

○   ○   **2. N = Neglected**
Have you ever neglected some of your usual daily responsibilities due to using sweets* or overeating?

○   ○   **3. C = Cut down**
Have you felt that you wanted or needed to cut down on eating sweets* in the last year?

○   ○   **4. O = Objected**
Has anyone objected to you overeating sweets*? Has your family, a friend, or anyone else ever told you they objected to, or were upset by, your eating habits?

○   ○   **5. P = Preoccupied**
Have you ever found yourself preoccupied with wanting sweets* or found yourself thinking a lot about sweets*?

○   ○   **6. E = Emotional discomfort**
Have you ever used sweets/food* to relieve emotional discomfort, such as fatigue, irritation, sadness, anger, tiredness or boredom?"

_____   **Number of Yes Answers**

Score of 0 or 1

You are a rare creature who can eat sugary foods in moderation. Keep an eye on your sugar and starchy carbohydrate intake to make sure it doesn't increase over time and keep eating nutrient dense foods.

Score of 2

Looks like there are some issues with your relationship to sugary foods. You may not have a full-blown addiction problem. Read on to learn more about carbohydrate addiction and the brain and be mindful of habitual or emotional eating of sugary foods.

Score of 3 to 6

This book is most certainly written for you. Welcome to the tribe. I'm sure you'll recognise yourself in many of the stories here. You are not alone in your struggles.

Which foods seem to be 'addictive'?

Not all foods are created equal when it comes to their addictive qualities. An American study in 2015 looked at which foods were 'problematic' for people. Not surprisingly, they were foods high in sugar and fat and those that were highly processed.

The Top Ten Offenders

1. Pizza
2. Chocolate
3. Crisps
4. Biscuits
5. Ice Cream
6. Chips
7. Cheeseburgers
8. Fizzy drinks
9. Cake
10. Cheese

Make a note of that last one because we will return to it in Chapter 3!

Chapter 1: Are You a Carbohydrate Addict?

Most carbohydrate addicts are more drawn to sweet things but I've met plenty of people who craved starchy and savoury foods such as bread and crisps, usually with plenty of butter.

A very important fact to understand, as I mentioned before, is that starchy foods high in carbohydrate such as bread, cereals, pasta and rice, digest down very quickly into glucose (sugar) in the body. So, an addiction to bread or pizza can still be understood as an addiction to sugar! Starch is sugar molecules holding hands!

Which foods are causing you most problems? Are they very sugary, starchy and fatty? What can you just not moderate and habitually overeat despite your best intentions? Are you able to stop at just one biscuit or square of milk chocolate? Being aware of exactly which foods are problematic for you is key to taking your fork in the road, perhaps make a list.

ANNA *I ate a whole bag of icing sugar mixed with water when I was pregnant with my first child. I was 18 and had quit using drugs when I found out I was pregnant. I felt ashamed because I knew it would harm my baby, but I needed a fix.*

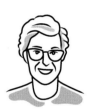

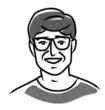

DAVE *I needed to eat several cookies before I got into the shower each morning. The shame of walking down to get them and having to walk back up the stairs with my fix before being able to start getting ready for work.*

BITTEN *I remember stealing "sugar lumps" (used in coffee in Sweden in the old days) from my grandmother's cabinet, I knew I was not allowed so was tiptoeing and being very quiet. I was 4-5 years old.*

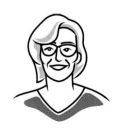

How can foods be addictive?

I like to look at this from an evolutionary perspective. The ability to overeat, especially in the autumn, was a matter of survival for most of our evolution. Carbohydrate rich foods like fruits and tubers were available before the winter and enabled us to put on fat to get through the winter. In this way it can be seen as adaptive that carbohydrate foods bypass the natural 'fullness' signalling we get from protein and fat, so we are able to eat more of them and for longer. Notice how you may be 'stuffed' after a huge dinner but can still manage pudding! We are highly motivated to seek out fattening foods. We are here today because our ancestors were very good at putting on fat in the autumn! We sugar addicts would be the best survivors.

Unfortunately, in our modern food environment this ability has become a liability! When high carbohydrate foods are everywhere, every day, instead of for a few weeks a year AND they are highly processed, then we have a big problem.

Food today is 'hyperpalatable', and designed to be that way, so that we eat more of it. Food scientists have literally studied the 'bliss' point of salt, sugar and fat that humans find irresistible.

We are eating more and more processed foods, with horrible consequences for our physical and mental health. Every day we are bombarded with 'fake food'; breakfast cereals, snack bars, crisps, packaged and pre-made meals stuffed with sugar, industrial vegetable oils and weird ingredients to extend shelf life. It's no wonder we have epidemics of chronic mental and physical illnesses. And yet this way of eating is 'normalised'. Just like the cigarette industry before them, the food industry spends countless millions on suppressing the anti-sugar message and funding favourable science.

Those of us who choose to eat real food and shun sugar and carbohydrates are seen as the unusual ones. Recovery requires a whole new attitude to nutrition. It helped me to get angry about the misinformation I had been 'fed' all my life. We don't need carbohydrates at all, saturated fat is not bad for us, salt is not the enemy and we don't need to eat little and often! In fact, I pretty much unlearned everything I thought I knew about the proper human diet.

The physiology of addiction

Because sweet foods are linked to ancient survival mechanisms, we are highly motivated to pursue them. Our brain re-wires a little bit every time we encounter them. The brain transmitter involved in motivation and reward is dopamine. The primitive reward centre in the brain lights up in response to sugar, releasing dopamine. If you don't believe me, just Google 'baby's first ice cream' and watch the 30 second video. We are then motivated to repeat the behaviours that led up to the dopamine release.

Your brain remembers the cues of smell, sounds and colours associated with getting 'the hit' and you are driven to repeat the experience in the presence of those cues.

At the same time, the brain also protects itself against these strangely high levels of dopamine by reducing the number of available receptors. Next time, you will need a bigger piece of cake or a second biscuit to get the same results. Also, I hope you can see that the brain reducing its dopamine receptors is definitely not a good thing over time. Low dopamine is implicated in depression, concentration and memory problems. Addicts focus more and more on getting their 'hit', but it becomes harder and harder. Then the focus becomes just getting through the day without withdrawal symptoms. There is also a tendency to reduce other interests and activities, so that life comes to focus around food and food thoughts. Sound familiar?

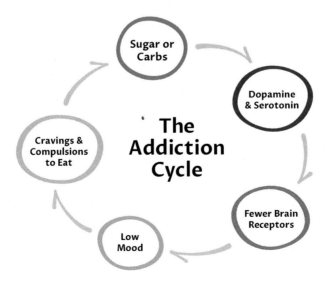

Dopamine is the reward and motivation transmitter whereas another chemical, serotonin signals comfort and wellbeing.
Antidepressants work by making serotonin more available in the brain. When we eat sugar and carbohydrate the body releases the hormone insulin from your pancreas gland. Insulin's job is to get sugar out of the bloodstream (where a raised blood sugar, as in type 2 diabetes, does damage over time) and into the muscle, liver and fat cells. When insulin is high (as after a carby meal or snack), tryptophan (an amino acid from food) can pass from the bloodstream into the brain more easily. Tryptophan is then converted into serotonin. So, in short, when we eat sugar, on top of the dopamine hit already described, we also get a boost of serotonin and a feeling of wellbeing and comfort. Most people recognise that sugary foods will lead to these feelings and can start to use food for emotional reasons. However, the brain will also down regulate serotonin receptors, meaning, over time, we need more sugar to get the same effect.

I hope you can see the desperate trap that carbohydrate addiction can become. We are left depleted emotionally at a biological level but also psychologically and behaviourally. People also suffer from aversive physical withdrawal symptoms when they can't access sugary foods. Shakiness, irritability, sleep problems, headache, fatigue and nausea are commonly experienced but resolve on consuming something high in carbohydrate. The sugar fix. Most people never go long enough to get through the withdrawal phase because of this. Another part of the trap!

The fact that sugar stimulates the survival and primitive parts of the brain means that your logical, thinking brain is overridden.

This is why we struggle to resist cravings with willpower. You need to act your way out of addiction over time with new habits, because you can't think your way out of it. As a psychologist I could never understand how I would decide not to eat biscuits in the morning but then helplessly watch my hand reaching for them in the afternoon. It wasn't my fault and it isn't yours. It is biology in action. This information will be your power.

GEORGIA *I never fully appreciated that food addiction was a big part of the problem until I got married after living alone for a long time. My partner noticed how preoccupied I was with food, how hard it was for me to resist overeating unless I followed my food plan to the letter, and how long it took me to get back on track after dietary indiscretions. Until that point, I had always viewed metabolic differences as my primary vulnerability.*

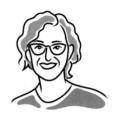

Hunger

Just getting back to the important hormone insulin, because of it's imperative to drive down blood sugars, 'the high' of eating that cookie is all too brief, with the crashing blood sugar levels come the feelings of hunger and even mild anxiety we experience as 'withdrawal'. We return to the cookie jar again in another miserable vicious cycle. Happily, this particular cycle does not have to be. We are in fact genius hybrid-engines built to burn two different fuels for energy; sugar and fat. Sadly, for the carb addicted amongst us the high levels of insulin block our ability to burn our (often ample) reserves of fat. So, when as a twelve stone teenager I so often felt ravenously hungry, insulin was to blame. Here we have another message of hope -the opposite of this is also true. A low carb diet enables us (after a period of adjustment) to become a fat burner -utilizing our fat reserves and feeling less hungry as a result! Stable blood sugars lead to stable moods and untold health benefits. The best diet for sugar addicts is also very healthy for the brain and body more generally.

The bottom line

If you ARE a carb addict then you will not be able to free yourself from the hold of certain foods unless you are able to truly acknowledge the addiction. Just like addiction to drugs, nicotine, alcohol or gambling, the bed rock of recovery is abstinence. That means that you have to come to the realisation that you are powerless to control your intake of certain foods. Moderation is not possible (because you've tried a thousand times), so the only option is to quit completely. **'Just one small piece', 'cheat day' or 'only at the weekend'** will NOT work for you. Ignore what other people say is possible! Moderation is a mythical unicorn to us. This isn't about a lack of willpower or a personal failing, it's about a physical and mental addiction. You are not to blame and abstinence will be your first step to freedom and brain healing. This acceptance is what I call the 'fork in the road' moment. The time you choose to follow a new path, the path to freedom from sugar and to living your best life. The road won't always be easy but it is the right road.

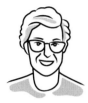

ANNA *Constant exposure to the "drug" is part of what triggers sugar/food addicts to relapse. Unlike other "things" (I don't have to be around drugs, or alcohol), I have to eat! Other people eat things that are psychoactive to me. It took me about six months to be completely abstaining from "drug foods".*

We all know people who aren't addicted to carbs, who can just have one biscuit, a small slice of cake or wave the dessert menu away after a meal.

But if you are reading this book, I'm guessing, like me, you're not one of them! They seem like alien creatures to us. Such people have no need to be fully abstinent from sugar. Some other people will habitually overeat sugar and refined carbohydrate out of habit and because it's so normal in our culture. They may be harming their health and could do with cutting down on sugary processed foods, but they are not sugar addicts. These 'harmful users' can also benefit from the information in this book. We carb addicts are a very special group, we need to follow certain rules to be free of cravings, obsessions and unwanted behaviours around food and weight.

DAVE

My sister was a sugar addict, my mother was a sugar addict. Apples do not fall far from trees, especially apple trees.

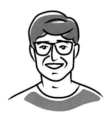

NEXT: Finding your motivation to give up your beloved drug foods.

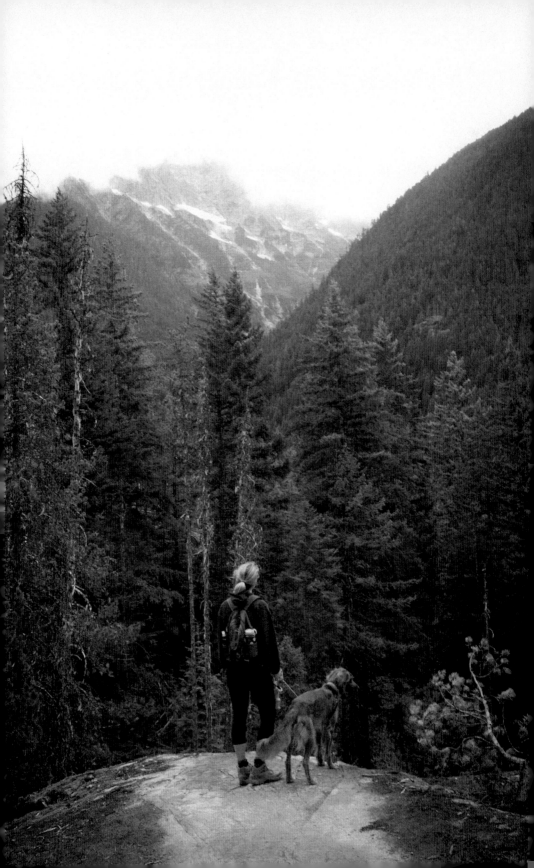

CHAPTER 2

Your Passport to Recovery

*The rules for recovery from carb addiction
are actually really, really simple.*

*No sugar, flour, processed foods.
No trigger foods.*

JEN *Recovery is simple but not easy. If it were easy, everyone would be doing it and food companies wouldn't be raking in the profits! It's not easy because your primitive brain will drive you and trick your willpower and logic at every turn to reach for those drug foods multiple times a day, particularly in the beginning.*

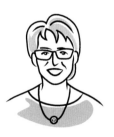

It does get easier, it really does. *But the first few days and weeks and even months will be a challenge. For that reason, you need all your motivation, hopes, strengths and resources with you from the start. You will stumble at times but I know you can get back up and try again because I did. Many others in recovery have walked this path before you.*

BITTEN *At menopause, 20 years ago, age 48, I had tried being abstinent but relapsed big time and panicked because I felt I could not stop eating chocolate, I gained weight, pain in my body, extreme fatigue and low on energy. Nothing was fun. It took me a long time to get back on the wagon with help from a professional.*

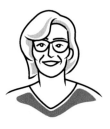

This chapter will help you to uncover all the mental strength you need to get back up and will be the foundation on which to build your food freedom. I'm going to use the analogy of a journey to help you explore your dream destination, what you need to take with you, your first stopover and keeping a travel log. These ideas have worked for me and the many people my husband David and I have worked with. You can apply the same thinking process to any life issue but here we will focus on your carb addiction journey.

Your dream destination

It can be easy to lose sight of our hopes and dreams when we get caught up in a problem like carb addiction. It can dominate our thoughts in a negative way and cause us to lose hope of a better future. The first task is to allow yourself to think about how you would like your carb-free life to look in six months, a year or five years from now. Don't think about how you would get there, just dream! Imagine you no longer had to think about food all the time, had ditched worries about weight, had a feeling of pride and control. You are finally free.

What could life look like then?

What would it liberate you to be able to do instead?

If your main goal is weight loss, what would losing weight allow you to achieve or what difference would it make in your life?

What do you notice yourself doing, feeling, and thinking in your happy weight and carb-free future?

What will other people notice about you?

What will be the first thing you notice when you wake up in the morning and the last thing you think before you go to bed?

Write down your thoughts or talk them through with someone who cares and understands. Get a clear image in your mind of you living your best life. In clinical practice we find the more someone is clear about their imagined future the more likely they are to achieve it!

A colleague of mine used to say 'it's a long day on the golf course if you don't know where the hole is'! You need a good idea of where you are heading if you are to stay on track for this long journey. I promise there will be a few wrong turns and miss hits along the way so you'd better know how to re-find your way back to your path!

Packing for your trip

What and who are you going to take on your recovery journey? You will need to pack your bag with all your best emergency supplies. Most of us have a long history of struggles with food and we have all dealt with a whole range of other life challenges by now. There are aspects of our characters that help us to deal with life and there maybe people who are on our side through thick and thin. Now is the time to gather all the useful resources you can and keep them close.

Have you had any times in your life when you were more in control of your carb addiction? What was going on then? A particular food plan? A phase of life that was easier? Something else? Reflecting on your journey to date can give you some hints at things you can keep doing or incorporate into your recovery. For example, I knew I could not have drug foods in the house and that I feel mentally stronger when I exercise regularly. Are there already things that are working well that you want to keep doing, such as taking a boxed lunch to work for example? What else?

Now don't be shy. What are your personal strengths and how can you use them? I've always been a very organised and timetabled person who loves routine and this is a great asset to recovery. If I set a grand plan in motion, I tend to stick to it. How about you? Determined, stubborn, organised, sociable? What would others say are your greatest character assets? How can they be brought to bear on your recovery journey? If you are struggling with this there is a free strengths test online. See Chapter 7.

What else helps you already? Or has in the past? I re-started yoga classes and spend my relaxing time knitting to keep my hands busy. If you aren't obsessed with food you will have some spare time on your hands. What will you use it for? *Much more on this issue in Chapter 5!*

Make a list of everything you want to keep in your suitcase.
There may be some things you want to ditch too as they will weigh you down or side track you!

First stop over

It might be a cheesy and overused phrase but the journey of a thousand miles truly does begin with the first step. Now you know where you are heading and what you already have in your suitcase you can plan your first leg of the trip! But what is to be your first step? The dream destination you have described is carb freedom and everything that will bring you. Assign it a 10/10 rating. The glorious future carb-free life is 10/10. You may be starting from zero or you may have already taken some steps. If you are not zero, what score out of 10 do you currently give yourself, and why? Then the next important question is how will you know that you have reached your first or next stop over? What would 1/10 (or 2/10 or 3/10, if you are not starting from zero) look like for you? How will you know that you have reached one small step closer to your goal? Or even half a step or a quarter step? A tiny step is still a start.

What would a tiny bit of progress look like for you?

_____

_____

What would tell you that you were making progress?

_____

_____

_____

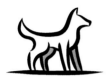 **Write it down. Tell your friend. Or your dog.**
In fact, what would the dog or friend notice that told them
something good was happening in your relationship to food?

**You won't think your way out of addiction, but you can
act your way out.**
Willpower is not a reliable friend. I once heard it said that it would be better
called won't power as you are usually trying not to do something! Better to slowly
build new habits. Once established, habits don't take much mental energy, they
become automatic, like brushing our teeth. Eventually you feel strange not doing
the behaviour.

So which small new habit will you try out?
Change your breakfast cereals for eggs?
Give up sugar in your hot drinks?
Quit fizzy drinks?
Biscuits?
*What feels attainable and
like a small step forward?*

**You may be planning on going all in on quitting carbs.
I can understand that because it is what I did.**
In which case please read the advice in Chapter 3: The Problem and the Remedy
before you start. Put in the advised preparation first. Do not embark immediately
on a low carbohydrate diet if you are taking diabetes or blood pressure medications or have chronic kidney or liver disease. Consult your doctor first in case
your medications need adjusting. There is plenty of reading and preparation
you can do in the meantime. Cupboards need clearing, food needs to be bought,
conversations with family and friends may need to happen.

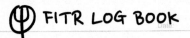 **FITR LOG BOOK**

You are embarking on your own journey into carb freedom.

Although the basic rules are the same for everyone, some will set out in a speed boat and others on foot!

The point of making changes and trying new things is to notice what works best for you personally. **There is no food plan that will suit everybody** so it's important to pay attention to your own wellbeing and progress. If you feel energetic without cravings, are maintaining a good weight and sleep well, then you are doing something right. If you are tired, hungry, worried and depressed then something else needs to change.

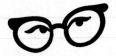 **KEEP PAYING ATTENTION**
to what works and keep doing that.
Then try another step forward.

EXPERIMENT WITH MEAL TIMINGS and sizes that fit around your routine. Some people like to keep an actual diary whereas others just take a mental note.

People around you can be a good guide too.
Ask them what they notice about you.
Are you more energetic? Less grumpy?

KINSHIP

So, what's important is that noticing what works for you provides feedback, and feedback is the bedrock of behaviour change. We are all so unique.

In clinical practice we use various tests to let people know how they are doing. It is possible blood pressure, diabetic control or liver function may improve for those who give up carbs, but give a thought to anything you can monitor at home. Perhaps your waist measurement, mood or weight?

I feel compelled to put a note in here about that famous instrument of mental torture: THE SCALES! May I suggest that you don't make them a central part of your life and recovery?

Weigh once a week at the same time if you must, but don't let the result cloud your week. There are many reasons for temporary weight increases, so don't be derailed by the scales. I gave them up totally for a couple of years, after realising there was never a result that helped. If the scales went up I felt deflated and disheartened (the enemy of the emotional eater) and if they went down I could justify eating more unnecessarily. I do weigh myself only once a week now but alongside other measures.

The tape measure is probably a better measure of progress, particularly if you measure around your belly button. Do this every week, it's a better indicator of metabolic health than weight or body mass index. Energy, mood, cravings and sleep are all worth tracking if you enjoy keeping records.

Recovery is a lifelong mission. What works will also change over time depending on your age, exercise levels, health, stress and so on. However you do it, it will pay to notice and review how you are doing and what progress you are making (or not) on a regular basis. It's particularly important to learn from mistakes and setbacks. These are actually our best teachers for sustained recovery. We return to this in Chapter 6. There is no such thing as failure on this journey. Just lessons learned and the finding of new paths forward. Every day you will have to make multiple choices around food, many forks in the road, so keep the destination in mind.

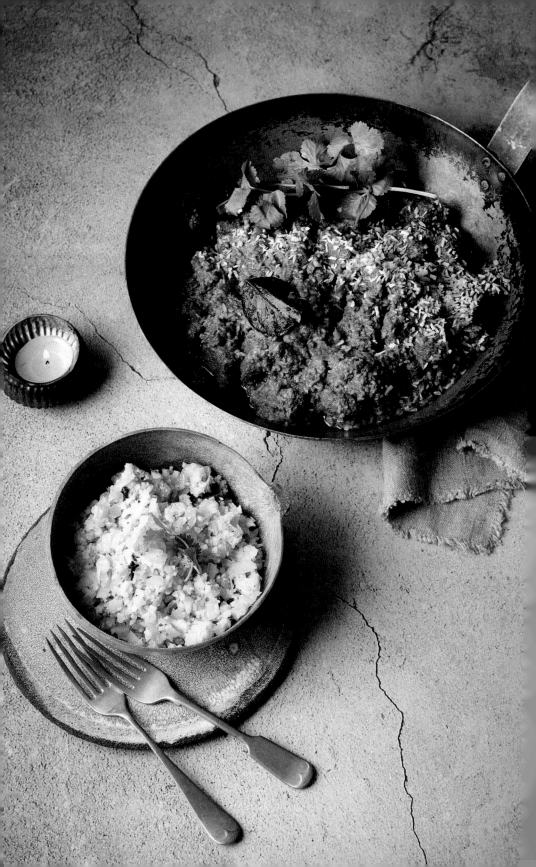

CHAPTER 3

The Problem and The Remedy

*Carbohydrate addiction is similar to
having a problem with nicotine or alcohol
but there is a big difference:
we have to eat.*

**People can give up cigarettes, drugs or alcohol and never 'need'
to pick them up again.** Other people admire and applaud you for giving
up those substances. Food is absolutely everywhere. It's at the paper shop till,
at the garage, at the office. Food and particularly carby foods are now central to
birthdays, Mother's Day, Easter, holidays, Valentines, Halloween, Christmas,
and weekends.

DAVE *As a dietician, I have seen food addicts come
into my office totally lost on what to do and how to
approach recovery from carb and food addiction.
If you focus on real foods, your cravings will have no
chance. I stand behind the advice here. I would offer it
to someone I loved. Please understand that food is a very small piece
of what recovery is, but if you follow this guidance you have made a huge
leap forward to a life of meaningful recovery. I am a food addict and have
worked with food addicts for over ten years. The food plans and principles
that work are beautifully outlined here.*

We have complex personal and family relationships with food

Food is culture, family, love and entertainment. Food is also essential. Carbs might just be the hardest drug to quit. Often, we get hooked as kids. Carby foods and junk foods are used as a reward, the very basis of the psychological mechanism of 'conditioning' (remember Pavlov's dogs?). Try to quit and we are mostly met with questions and pushback from friends and family rather than understanding and support.

In the world of addiction there is also some commonality. How often do people who give up alcohol and cigarettes start craving sweets and snacks? Even people who have bariatric surgery can end up putting the weight back on eventually or turning to alcohol. Yet others of us may be addicted to foods, nicotine and alcohol. David and I have been helping a young man who was addicted to sugar, nicotine, marijuana, alcohol and gaming. He noticed what worked with his sugar and carb addiction first and then repeated the process to eliminate first cigarettes, then alcohol, marijuana, and gaming. He has lost over 110 lbs and taken up running. Success can breed more success!

We are bombarded with conflicting nutrition advice

Fat is bad/good, meat is good/bad, carbs are good/bad, dairy is good/bad, eat frequently/infrequently, salt is good/bad etc. I can remember thinking if some-one would just tell me what to eat, when and how much. I was at a loss. A mass of confusion and hopelessness. This is why the 'shake' diets are superficially appealing. They take the doubt out of eating for a while. The problem is that you can't live on them forever and they are full of processed and fake ingredients.

Our approach is to eliminate all the foods that prevent you from being able to listen to your own natural hunger and fullness signals

Animals in the wild don't have to go on diets because they eat when hungry and stop when full. Natural whole foods, high in protein and fat, send signals to the brain to stop eating. You will be feeding your body what it needs to thrive. Carby and processed foods override natural fullness signals. As I mentioned earlier there is no 'off switch' for sugar and starchy carbs for so many of us. Unfortunately, that leads to physical and mental harm in the long run. Sugar and other processed foods cause damage and inflammation in the body leading to chronic health problems like type 2 diabetes, fatigue, mental health problems, digestive issues, headaches etc., etc.

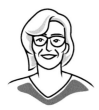

BITTEN *In 1993 I asked the program director I worked with on chemical dependency, from Chicago, why I had such a battle giving up sugar. I told her I had quit drinking, I am a recovering alcoholic since 1985, and quit smoking in 1992. She said you might be a food addict.*
I understood addiction but could not see that food could be addictive. When that started to sink in, I was shocked and very sad, I did not want to give up carbs at all but part of me knew I had to if I wanted to stay in recovery. I also learned that sugar is a risk factor in relapsing with alcohol. I also could see that my addictions started with sugar and progressed to nicotine and then alcohol. It became very clear.

Some important physiology

Part of the problem with dietary carbohydrates concerns its relationship to the hormone insulin, produced by the pancreas gland. As we have learnt from those with diabetes, a high blood sugar damages over time the lining of our arteries. (This is why people with poorly controlled diabetes get heart, eye and kidney problems.) We are cleverly designed so that our insulin pushes sugar from the blood where it is dangerous, to inside our cells to provide energy. For muscle cells the need for this energy is obvious. But what if you consume more sugar than needed by your muscles? In this case your body still has the imperative to get the sugar out of the bloodstream, fast! Now insulin pushes the blood sugar into other cells; those in the liver and abdomen. Because the sugar is not needed, it is stored for future use as fat. Causing big tummies and fatty liver.

Non-alcoholic fatty liver as it is more properly called now affects 20% of the developed world, unfortunately it adversely affects health in many ways, for instance it reduces your sensitivity to insulin itself, so helping to usher in diabetes and high blood pressure.

The great news is that human beings have ZERO requirement for carbohydrate in their diet

We do need a small amount of blood glucose (about a teaspoon in the whole body) but we can make it ourselves from protein and fat in the liver. This is why humans have survived periods of starvation. It is FALSE that we need carbohydrate or sugar for energy. That is marketing not science. David and I have been on a super low carbohydrate diet for over seven years now and I run three times a week and do weights three times a week. The essential nutrients for life and health are protein and fat. You don't need carbs and junk food. You might want it because your brain tells you so but maybe life without it will be all the more delicious and certainly healthier.

Becoming a fat burner and less hungry

You may not have realised but we are a dual-fuel engine, rather like the new hybrid cars. We can actually burn either sugar (glucose) or fat for energy. I mentioned earlier about insulin's imperative to drive blood sugar down. As part of this Insulin also blocks fat burning – it wants you to burn sugar first. However, once the sugar in your diet has been dealt with, say overnight, insulin drops allowing you to burn your reserves of fat. This explains the basis of the so called 'keto diet'. If dietary sugars and all sources of sugar (more on this later) are low, much less insulin is needed, so insulin levels drop, allowing fat burning to take over as the major fuel source. Much of this centres on the liver which converts fat into ketones (as in 'nutritional ketosis' or being 'keto'), an excellent fuel.

To become a maximum fat burner can take up to two weeks

But it has several advantages. Firstly, you are better able to access and burn your own fat stores which could help with weight loss. In our low carb clinics the average patient loses about 9kg (20lbs) in weight. The greatest loss so far has been over 10 stone (64 kgs/140 lbs)! Also, this is how you can avoid any need for dietary carbohydrates. Finally, hunger is in part a warning that you are getting low on fuel. Most of us carry weeks of energy reserves as fat so once you are a fat burner hunger is far less of a problem. The commonest observation of those on a low carb diet is how surprised they are not to be hungry. David hears this in every clinic, indeed he often recounts how he was hungry all his life until he went low carb in December 2012. Now he manages happily on one or two meals a day. This lessening of hunger can be very helpful to us in avoiding making poor, impulsive food choices.

Food for thought

Ingredient list for a popular doughnut brand.

DOUGHNUT
Enriched Wheat Flour: Wheat Flour, Niacin, Reduced Iron, Thiamine
Monoitrate, Riboflavin, Folic Acid], Water, Palm Oil, Soybean Oil, Sugar.
Contains 2% or less of each of the following: Yeast, Soy Lecithin,
Hydrogenated Soybean Oil, Mono and Diglycerides, Salt, Wheat Gluten,
Monocalcium Phosphate Monohydrate, BHT, Dried Milk Power, Egg Yolks,
Cellulose Gum, Calcium Propionate (to maintain fressness), Lecithin,
Oat Fiber, Ascorbic Acid, Sorbitan Monostearate, Tocopherols).
Glaze: Sugar, Water, Corn Starch, Palm Oil, Calcium Sulfate and/or
Calcium Carbonate, Agar, Destrose, Natural and Artificial Flavors, Salt,
Disodium Phosphate, Locust Bean Gum and/or Mono and Diglycerides.

Recovery comes when we abstain from the foods that trigger cravings and overeating

You will need to experiment to find the exact right foods, amounts and timings
for you but many recovering carb addicts will agree with the basic principle of
abstinence from sugar and flour to get you started and free of the white stuff.
This advice is for people with a history of the symptoms of food addiction, not
for people who can moderate what they eat (lucky them!).

Think of someone trying to give up alcohol or cigarettes, should they try just a small whiskey or half a cigarette?

Unfortunately, in order to succeed many of us have to face up to abstinence
from the things we crave. Bear in mind if you are on long term medications,
particularly for diabetes, it is very important that you consult your healthcare
provider if you have any long-term health conditions before you change
your diet.

Remember it may be the foods you feel you 'cannot live without' that are the very
ones you should let go. In clinical practice we notice some people have feelings of
panic at even the idea of giving up their problem foods. We've had people in tears
about their relationship with bread.

Think of these as NOT food

Always, and as soon as possible, abstain from these foods.

Sugar Eating sugar releases dopamine in our bodies. Dopamine is a neurotransmitter that is a key part of the "reward circuit" associated with addictive behavior.

Sweeteners These can lead to cravings and keep the 'sweet tooth' going. If you need them as a transition from sugar that's ok but keep in mind that you need to quit them eventually.

Flour Bread cakes or biscuits.

Breakfast cereals Cereals are loaded with refined grains, sugar, preservatives, artificial sweeteners, and other ingredients.

Junk Food Nearly always a combination of refined carbohydrates, fat and salt (pizza, burgers, doughnuts) not to mention a host of weird chemicals.

Alcohol Many alcoholic drinks are sugar-based and alcohol acts in the same area of the brain as sugar, making it easier to relapse.

Foods to abstain from or be very cautious with

Dairy Milk, cream, cheese are commonly craved by food addicts.

Nuts and Seeds Commonly overeaten and craved by food addicts.

Higher sugar fruits Modern fruits like bananas have much more sugar in them. (6 teaspoons on average!)

Caffeine Some food addicts do better cutting out caffeine.

What is left is our proper ancestral human diet

Real, whole-foods: meat, fish, eggs, fats, low-sugar fruits and green vegetables. Things that don't come in packages. Think about these foods. In my experience these 'whole foods' are never the source of cravings or addiction. You may really enjoy a big steak and salad but it will quickly fill you up quite unlike ice-cream, biscuits or trifle! Study the food lists on page 54 for more details.

Low carb gives you food freedom

GEORGIA *A typical day for me might include salmon, duck breast, chicken broth, seltzer, one small cup of coffee or tea, and occasionally a few low-carb plant foods that don't seem to bother me such as cucumber, zucchini, olives, or mushrooms. I usually eat between noon and 6 PM.*

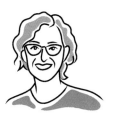

Starchy carbohydrate foods like rice, potatoes or bread are actually high-sugar foods when they are dealt with in the body by digestion. In fact, the starch molecule is glucose molecules joined together that your digestion will split back down into sugar again. So just because it isn't sweet doesn't mean it won't set off cravings. Look at just how much sugar is in some common foods. This isn't just a problem from a carb addiction point of view. Excess carbohydrate leads to high insulin which causes fat storage and ultimately metabolic problems leading to serious long-term conditions such as diabetes and heart disease. Alzheimer's, several cancers and other serious conditions have also been linked to poor metabolic health and obesity — common in those with a poor diet.

I know some of you will already be thinking that it isn't possible to live only on the green list foods

I would have thought that once too. But now I know the freedom that comes with this lifestyle far outweighs the momentary pleasure of a cupcake or chocolate bar. The kind of food plan you are aiming for is often referred to as low carbohydrate or keto. Many of you will have tried such plans before and eventually 'failed'. I did Atkins for a few years and did really well until I started eating more processed meats and snacks and eventually relapsed. Many keto and low carb plans allow high levels of dairy or have whole books on recreating breads, cakes and 'junk food'. I'm not certain of many things, but I know our ancestors were not eating cupcakes made with nut flours and sweetener! I have made these things in the past but it always ended badly. You are aiming for a very clean keto or low carbohydrate plan.

There are two ways to transition to a new food plan

Either 'cold turkey' or step wise. Both require a great deal of planning and determination. Go with what is right for you and if it doesn't work try another way. I went cold turkey initially but have also worked hard on a range of habits over the years like sticking to black decaff coffee, giving up the idea of dark chocolate and nuts, eating less frequently and finally quitting alcohol this year. Think of it as lifelong self-improvement. The advantage of cold turkey is that it takes the complexity out of transition and after a few days you will get to feel the glorious benefits of being free of drug foods. My husband, David, did it in a more stepwise way but he isn't really a full-blown carb addict. He had a bad biscuit habit, it sounds ridiculous but they were part of how he coped with being senior partner at the practice. To make giving them up possible, he transitioned from Jaffa Cakes to plain oat biscuits and then onto almonds, after a year he was able to stop snacking all together. However, the downside for anyone 'transitioning' is that they are vulnerable to slipping back during the process.

Preparing for your successful new way of eating

In the early days of recovery, you will be very vulnerable to cravings and temptation. Be prepared by doing everything you can to maximise your chances of getting at least two weeks of sugar-, flour- and grain-free eating under your belt. By that stage the majority of people will be noticing the upsides of giving up these foods. Brighter mood, more energy, better sleep and so on. Noticing these benefits will help you to keep going and get you back on track if you sway.

1. **Set a date to start.** Choose a time without too many big commitments, socialising or disruption but not a two-week holiday as its actually good to keep your mind busy.

2. **Go through your cupboards, fridge and freezer in advance and get rid of all your 'drug' foods.** From now on you are eating for health, not for amusement. Give stuff away, donate to the food bank or bin it. The bin is where that stuff belongs, not in you. You are not a dustbin. I do get that people hate food waste though, so give it away if you can't bin it.

3. **Re-stock your fridge, freezer and cupboards with recovery foods from the green list.** Some tins and jars are fine but ALWAYS read the label to check for SUGAR. Its everywhere. Find local sources of quality fresh vegetables, meat and fish. You will be saving the planet as well as yourself by not eating food flown around the planet and it works out cheaper. Consider shopping online for bulk items so you don't need to be tempted at the supermarket.

4. **Have your own cupboard, fridge shelf and freezer section** if other people in the house are not going to follow the same nutrition plan as you. The idea is to look as little as possible at trigger foods in the first few weeks. I can now happily go to buffets and walk straight past the chips, sandwiches, cakes and deserts. In the early days I would have been unable to do that.

5. **Discuss with house mates and family what you are doing and why.** It will depend on your circumstances whether you will be cooking for yourself or still catering for others. I used to make the main meal e.g., chicken curry and green beans then add microwave rice for my son who was still having carbs at that point. Keep it simple.

6. **Plan your eating, particularly at first.** Make sure you have plenty of tasty and nutritious real food so as not to be hungry. Fat is allowed and necessary for recovery. This is not a DIET. It's a way of life.

7. **Start with three good meals a day based on protein, veg/salad and good fats.** Have breakfast when you get hungry, if you never ate it, no need to start now, just have two good meals a day. Don't eat after 6pm. This is much better for your metabolism.

8. **Try not to snack,** but if you need to, choose something high in protein/fat.

9. **Some people who cut back hard on carbs get a thing called 'keto-flu'** for a few days. This may include; headaches, mild nausea, poor concentration and muscle cramps. It is due to the body changing over to fat burning as described earlier. It helps to stay hydrated, avoid strenuous exercise, and increase dietary salt (the lower insulin levels cause you to wee out a lot of salt).

10. **If you are on prescribed medication particularly for diabetes your plan will need checking with the doctor or nurse** responsible in case doses need to change.

I've given an example day of eating just as a loose guide. It's important that you eat the foods you like. Also notice when you are truly hungry rather than eating out of habit. Many of us on low carbohydrate diets find that after a few weeks we are much less hungry and drop snacks and sometimes meals. I never eat breakfast now. I never snack. I have a big lunch. Find what works best for you and your schedule.

⚇ Fork in the Road **Food Guide**

E A T & E N J O Y

Treat yourself to the best you can afford: organic, free-range, grass-fed.
You will also be saving money by not eating junk and take outs.

Beef, Lamb & Pork
Choose sausages with high meat
content and no added sugar

Eggs, Chicken, Duck & Turkey

Fish & Shellfish
Including quality canned tuna

Game Meats
Bison, Goose, Elk, Rabbit,
Pheasant & Ostrich

Offal
Bone Marrow, Kidney,
Tongue, Liver & Heart

Lard & Tallow
Pork & Beef Fat

Butter & Ghee

Oils
Olive & Avocado Oil
Coconut Oil

Mustard & Mayonnaise
Avoid mayo made with vegetable oils.
Make your own.

Above-Ground Veggies
Cabbage, Cauliflower, Broccoli,
Courgette/Zucchini, Onions,
& Green Beans

Vegetable & Green Salads
Careful, dressings are often
loaded with sugar

Avocados & Olives

Sauerkraut & Pickles
Check labels for sugar.
Make your own.

Herbs & Spices
Fresh Ginger & Garlic

Lemon & Lime

Carbonated & Still Water
Add a squeeze of lemon, lime
or cucumber

Coffee & Tea
Coffee with no sugar or sweeteners
Herb & Fruit Tea, Black Tea
Ideally decaffeinated

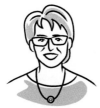

*"A low-carb way of eating is
not a deprivation diet, but rather
a celebration of a life eating
delicious food."*
DR JEN UNWIN

FORK IN THE ROAD

VENTURE WITH CAUTION

Add to the abstain list if you tend to overeat these

Starchy Vegetables
Potatoes, Peas, Sweetcorn,
Sweet Potato, Beetroot & Carrot

Legumes & Beans
Can cause bloating for some folks.

Nightshades
Tomatoes, Eggplant & Peppers

**Apples, Peaches, Melons,
Pears & Berries**

Bacon, Salami & Cured Meats
Check labels for sugar

Almond & Coconut Flour

90% Dark Chocolate

Nuts & Seeds
Especially salted

Nut Butters
Peanut, Almond & Cashew

Full-Fat Greek Yoghurt

Cream & Milk
Cream has less sugar than milk in coffee.
Dairy is problematic for some people.
Goat and sheep milk can be better.

Cheese

ABSTAIN & REFRAIN

This can seem daunting at first, but becomes normal with time

Refined Table Sugar

Natural Sugars
Honey & Maple Syrup

Sweeteners
Alcohol & Artificial

Vegetable & Seed Oils
Margarine, Canola (Rapeseed) Oil,
Sunflower & Safflower Oil

Alcohol

Sugary Drinks
Soda Pop, Apple & Orange Juice

Fake Milks
Soy, Rice & Oat Milk

Grains & Starches
Bread, Rice, Potatoes,
Pasta, Crisps & Chips

**Biscuits/Cookies
Pastry, Cakes & Candy**

**Smoothies, Ice Cream
& Low-Fat Yoghurt**

Tropical Fruit
Bananas, Pineapple & Mangoes

**Dried Fruit,
Raisins & Grapes**

Ketchup
Condiments with Sugar

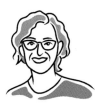 **GEORGIA** *For me (and for quite a few of my patients as well), sugar is not the issue; starches, dairy, and even intensely seasoned whole foods are the things that trigger cravings and overeating. Many of my patients had already tried completely eliminating sugar from their lives but noticed no improvement of any kind in their mental or physical health. It doesn't have to be sweet to be addictive.*

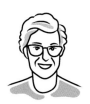 **ANNA** *I applied my program, stayed honest, and learned from my relapses that one lick, one smidgeon, one crumb, releases the obsession to use all over again. I like being food sober, my mind is clear, and I am free, so I tell myself on a daily basis sugar is poison, it is not harmless, I visualize skull and crossbones on "drug foods" when I see them or even when I smell them. I don't eat drug foods. Feelings cannot be eaten. Food has never "fixed" anything.*

DAVE *I play the tape through in my head. What will happen if I try just one… What always happens is I feel guilty, knew better than this and I feel alone and frustrated. I beat myself up. If I focus on what really happens if I eat one of my triggers I am able to steer clear because I know I am only abandoning myself, my health and my recovery.*

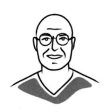 **MICHAEL** *Visuals are a big part of the triggering process for me. It starts at the grocery store: there is an entire aisle (of desserts) at Trader Joe's I just don't go to. Sometimes, especially around holidays, sweets make it into our home. I immediately get them off the kitchen counter and tuck them away in a drawer or cabinet so they are out of sight.*

EATING FOR RECOVERY - A TYPICAL DAY

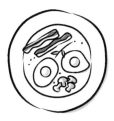 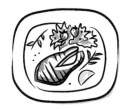 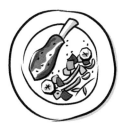

Breakfast	**Lunch**	**Dinner**
Bacon, 2 or 3 eggs, and mushrooms or scrambled eggs with butter	Fish (200g) with a salad or veggies and dressing *Grilled Salmon (pg 69)*	Meat (200g) with veggies and sauce *Slow-Cook Lamb Shanks (pg 87)*

The amounts are not rules

This isn't a diet. If you are very active, male and tall you will need more protein and fat. You should be able to go to the next meal without snacking. If you are struggling between meals initially have a high protein snack like hard boiled eggs or slices of ham. Drink plenty of fluid. Particularly in the early days you will need more salt as explained earlier so add plenty to your food.

Take food to work and when you travel so you know there won't be a panic. I used to take two raw eggs, a few cherry tomatoes and a cube of butter to work in a food box and microwave it when I got there. I also took leftovers to re-heat for lunch or a big boxed up salad with plenty of protein and dressing. When traveling we have taken pre-cooked and cooled pork belly slices on the airplane. In this way you won't be tempted by the ubiquitous sandwich and crisps options.

When going to other people's houses try and let them know you don't eat carbs and sugar before you go. It makes it easier on the day. If it's a party or buffet, make sure you take food you can eat and don't go very hungry beforehand. Maybe a cold meat/smoked salmon plate? Egg mayonnaise? Crudités with dips?

Chapter 3 : The Problem and The Remedy

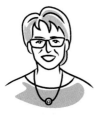 **JEN** *People will not always understand or want to understand. Have the conviction to stand your ground and leave if you have to. Have an exit strategy. Always have a back up plan. Eating out is something I've always loved. I've just adapted how I order. If bread is brought to the table, say you don't want it. It's hard to resist once it's there. We ask to keep the butter to add to our food! Choose your meal to be as compliant as you can. Prawn salad, pate, charcuterie to start for example. Meat or fish with vegetables for main course. Steak is perfect. If you aren't full after that we have been known to have another starter instead of the pudding! Or have the cheese course if it doesn't kick off cravings for you.*

We have never had an issue with special requests. Of course, certain places are more of a challenge and we don't go to Chinese restaurants now because many of the sauces have sugar in. In an Indian restaurant choose the mixed tandoori with vegetable sides. Most of all, learn to love your kitchen and get cooking!

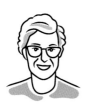 **ANNA** *I eat beef, seafood, poultry, pork, eggs, bone marrow, cod liver, butter, some cheeses, yogurt, cottage cheese etc. I use mostly animal fats for eating and cooking. I have fermented veggies like pickles and kraut occasionally, and a serving of veggies once in a while. I have five auto-immune conditions, and my RA (rheumatoid arthritis) is in complete remission right now, so it is easy for me to eat this way, not a punishment. Each bite I eat, I enjoy. I know I am providing my body with deep nutrition. I don't worry about what others think or about what they eat. This is my food plan and it works for me. I eat to satiety, and do not weigh or measure. I do not think everyone has to eat "my way". Each person must find a food plan that works for them.*

GEORGIA *While low glycaemic index diets, low-carbo-hydrate diets, exercise, and portion control all helped with recovery efforts to some extent over the years, I credit a lecture by Dr. Ron Rosedale for opening my eyes to the benefits of protein moderation. It was really the* 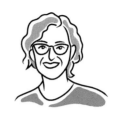 *discovery of the concept of ketosis (which was harder for me to achieve with carbohydrate restriction alone) that allowed me to experience significant and sustainable relief from cravings for the first time.*

BITTEN *My typical day is: 5-6 AM Bulletproof Coffee, water, midday protein (meat any kind, eggs, fish), fat (usually butter or ghee) and sometimes above ground veggies, such as cooked broccoli. Mid-afternoon, water and one cup decaf, sometimes with MCT oil and collagen. 5-6 PM the same as lunch.*

DAVE *My food plan is simple: primarily meat and low carbohydrate vegeta-bles. Fat for cooking. Drinks: decaffeinated tea and black coffee. Nothing complex about it. I love to cook, but even more I love to keep it simple. I have been known to eat a big ground beef patty, seasoned with salt and a splash of sugar-free hot sauce or to eat six eggs cooked in grass-fed butter.*

———————— IMPORTANT ————————

If you are taking medication it is really important that you consult with your health professional before starting to reduce sugar and carbohydrate in your diet.

Your doses may need adjusting or some medications may need stopping. In the first couple of weeks the following can be experienced; headaches, light-headed-ness, shaking, fatigue, poor sleep, gastric changes. Do not take vigorous exercise during this time. Increase the salt in your diet and have a salt shot or take electro-lytes if you have these symptoms. Some people may benefit from a magnesium supplement. Your body is shifting from sugar to fat for fuel and it takes some days to adjust. Most people feel better in a week or so and continue to improve in terms of exercise.

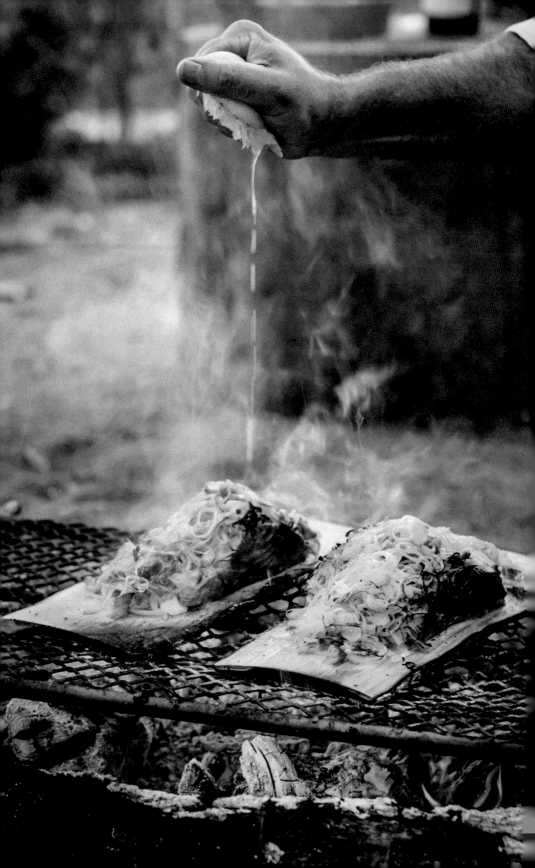

CHAPTER 4

Recipes

*Many sugar addicts are foodies.
We love to eat but we also love to cook,
go to restaurants, and talk about food
all day long. This is part of my life.
I am definitely not willing to give it up.*

My love of cooking is an advantage because I am able to understand recipes and cooking techniques and can make my meals delicious but sugar and carbohydrate free. I still get enormous pleasure from cooking and eating but without the downsides of guilt, weight gain and obsessing about what I have eaten, will or won't eat next. The day I understood that fat wasn't my enemy but part of my salvation was a great day. Fat makes everything delicious.

I couldn't believe fatty meat was back on the menu. It is what I eat most days now. Slow cooking and roasts are so easy and also if you make extra you can freeze it or eat it the next day.

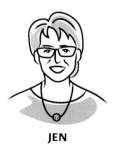

JEN

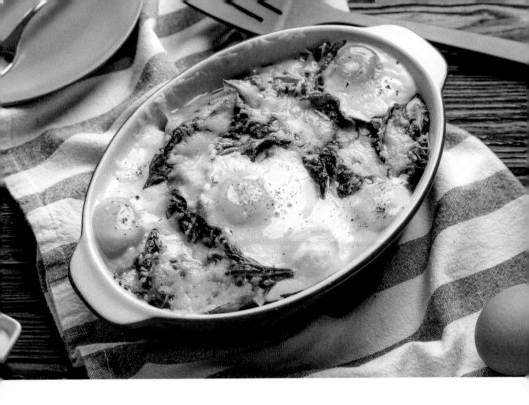

Eggs

Eggs, nature's super food. So easy, delicious and nutritious. Boiled eggs, fried eggs, scrambled eggs or omelettes are great. And don't forget egg mayonnaise. Add olive oil, butter or ghee for cooking. Get quality salt and pepper. Add herbs.

Useful for breakfast or lunch, good in salads. Even portable if you pre-boil and cool them. Our frittata recipe is great for any meal. You can eat it cold at work too with salad. Don't feel you have to stick to our recipe. Add your favourite flavours or just what's in your fridge. Add some cheese if you are okay with dairy.

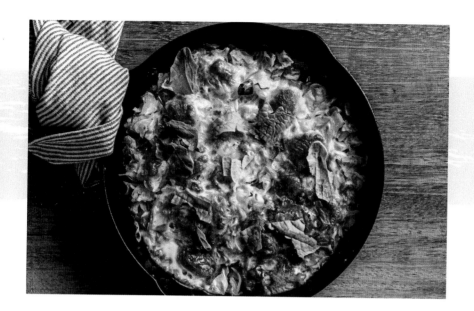

Frittata

6 eggs (*organic if you have them*)
chives *or other fresh/dried herbs*
A finely chopped red onion
A finely chopped red pepper

chopped chorizo,
or pancetta or bacon
olive oil, lard or ghee
salt and pepper

Heat a tablespoon of fat in an oven proof frying pan. Fry the chorizo and/or bacon for a few minutes until browning.

Add the chopped onion and fry until also a little caramelised. Add the pepper and fry. Take off the heat to cool. Beat up the eggs and chopped herbs in a bowl.

Add seasoning. Add to the cooled onion and pepper etc and stir. You can cook it under the grill or in a hot oven for 5 to 10 minutes.

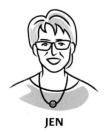

So versatile: salmon and asparagus, spinach, mushroom, sausage, avocado, ham, pesto, courgette, prawns, are all possibilities. For a portable snack or breakfast, bake in a bun tin to make mini versions. Children love them.

JEN

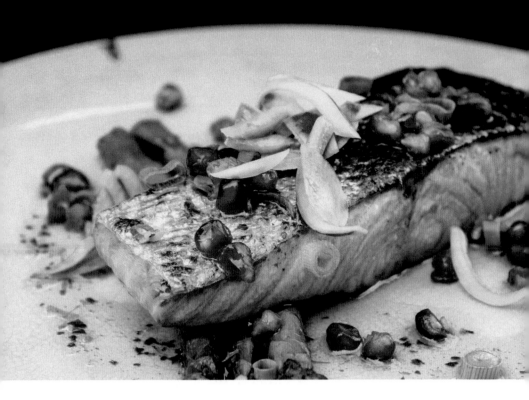

Fish

Fish is a healthy option. More brain food.
If you don't like to cook it, choose it in restaurants.

Quality tinned tuna in olive oil or defrosted cooked prawns
can make a quick nutritious lunch mixed into mayonnaise with salad.
Add some boiled eggs. For some, tinned sardines are an acquired taste,
but they are very nutritious! Smoked salmon, especially if wild caught,
is a treat. No cooking skills needed. Cooking fish is quick and simple.
Bake in the oven, fry in butter, or grill. No need to complicate things!
Serve with garlic butter, herb sauce, hollandaise,
or pesto from the options here.

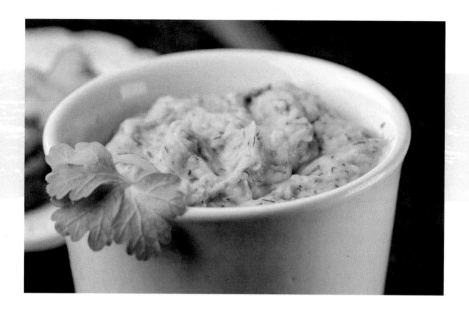

Smoked Mackerel Pate

Smoked mackerel is cheap and keeps well, this pate is quick to make and can be served as a lunch or starter.

200g smoked mackerel
— *skin removed and flaked*
150g melted butter *or ghee*
50g sour cream or yoghurt *(optional)*

1 tsp Dijon mustard
1 tbsp fresh parsley
juice and zest of a lemon

Mix everything together in a bowl with a fork.
Season to taste. Chill.

Cod sauteed in butter with salt and white pepper and an egg sauce. The sauce is hardboiled eggs, chopped, in lots of melted butter and lots of horseradish. I often eat this with some boiled broccoli or garlic butter-sauteed haricots verts. I never read recipes. I cook freestyle!

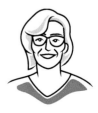

BITTEN

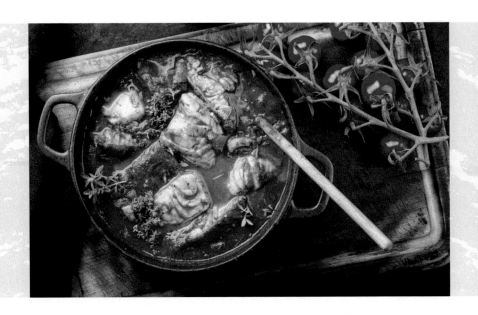

Marek Sumesh Fish Stew

This Kuwaiti dish is an easy and delicious fish stew that fills my kitchen with the exotic aroma of the Middle East. It is traditionally made with black dried lemons; they have a wonderful umami, citrus flavour and are available at Middle Eastern shops.

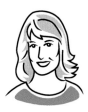

KATIE

This is our friend Amal's recipe who brings us a whole suitcase of black lemons, juicy dates and bags of spice from her local Souk every time she visits. Black lemons make your mouth pucker when you bite into them similar to preserved lemons so you can use those instead in a smaller quantity.

Umami = Delicious

SERVES 6
1 medium brown or white onion, *finely chopped*
5 tbsp of olive oil
2 cloves garlic, *peeled and finely chopped*
half to 1 hot chilli, *finely chopped, added according to taste*
salt and freshly-ground black pepper
1 tsp turmeric powder
1 tsp cumin
½ tsp coriander (cilantro) powder
25g fresh coriander (cilantro), *finely chopped — stalks and all*
2 x 400g tin of plum tomatoes
2 tbsp tomato concentrate
3 black dried lemons *or 1 tablespoon of preserved lemons, finely diced*
1 cod (or similar white fish) fillet, *about 800g, cut into portions*

FOR THE FISH
1 tsp turmeric
2 tsp ground cumin
1 tsp black pepper
2 tbsp olive oil or ghee *for frying*
salt

Cook the onion, garlic and chilli with seasoning in the oil until soft in a large wide pan over a gentle heat. Add the tomatoes and wash out the cans with about 150ml water and add this too. Mash the tomatoes with a potato masher and bring to a gentle boil. Heat through and add spices and pepper, fresh coriander, lemons and stir through.

Cook for about half an hour or until you have a thick sauce.

Mix the turmeric with cumin and black pepper on a large plate. **Season the fish with salt and rub the spice mixture evenly into the pieces of fish.** Heat the oil in a large frying pan and fry the fish over a gentle heat for a couple of minutes a side until lightly browned. Carefully transfer to the pan with the tomato sauce.

Continue to cook for around 15 minutes or until the fish is cooked through. Serve with cauliflower rice or on its own in soup bowls.

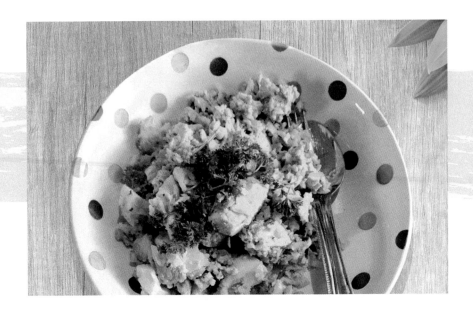

Kedgeree

This was one of my favourite meals as a child. It's quite easy to make it low carb.

200g smoked haddock
500g cauliflower
riced or very finely chopped
2 eggs-boiled, *shelled and quartered*
2 tbsp fresh parsley

2 tsp curry powder
2 tsp mustard
1-2 tbsp butter *or ghee*
juice of half a lemon
salt and pepper

Bake or simmer the fish gently in water or milk for 5-6 minutes until it flakes with a fork into small chunks. Drain. Melt the butter in a large pan. Add the spices and mustard. Stir.

JEN

Add the riced cauliflower. Add half a glass of the fish water/milk or stock and simmer for 5 minutes. Keep stirring.

On a gentle heat add the fish and stir. Simmer for another 5 minutes with the lid on. Add the lemon juice, salt and pepper to taste, parsley and stir. Transfer to a warm serving dish, top with boiled eggs and extra parsley.

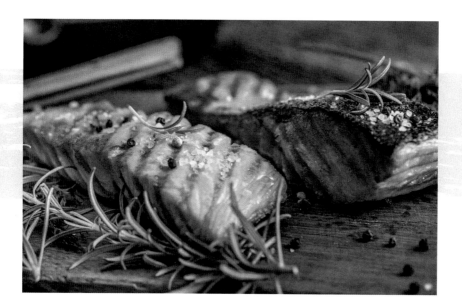

Grilled Salmon

wild-caught salmon	slices of lemon
coho, king, or sockeye	sprigs of rosemary
Half- to 1-pound per person	black pepper
olive oil	*or lemon pepper*

Drying and lightly oiling the salmon helps keep it from sticking to the grill. **Cover fish with olive oil, salt, and seasonings.** Allow it to come to room temperature before grilling.

Cleaning and oiling the grill helps keep the fish from stick to the grill. **Heat the grill before putting on the fish on.**

Most of the cooking happens on the skin side, with the skin crisping and acting as an insulator of the delicate flesh. Grill until the fish exudes a milky white fat about 2-3 minutes. Then grill a final minute or so on the other side to finish.

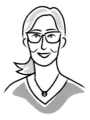

KIKI

Avoid Farm-Raised Fish
They are often fed an artificial diet and contain less nutrients than wild-caught. Previously frozen fish is fine.

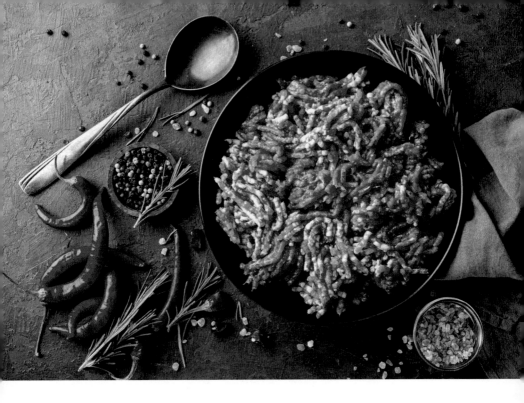

Mince

Cheap and versatile. Fatty minces (20%) are cheaper than lean minces and more satisfying. Use beef, pork or lamb mince. Combine beef with pork or lamb when making Bolognese or burgers.

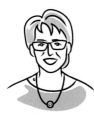

JEN

For easy meatballs and burgers, simply mix your required herbs, spices and seasoning into the mince with your hands. I often add mustard at this point. Shape, then fry or bake until cooked through. Serve with ratatouille, salad ,or celeriac chips and mayonnaise. You can use the basic Bolognese recipe to make low carb moussaka, lasagne or shepherd's pie. I use aubergine or courgette slices instead of pasta in a lasagne, I've also seen it done with blanched sheets of leek or swede. You can make a pie topping from celeriac or cauliflower mash. Add kidney beans to make a chilli. Buy organic, outdoor bred and grass-fed meats.

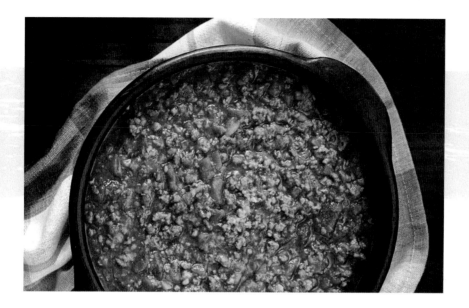

Bolognese

400g mince (ground beef)
4 tbsp olive oil
chopped bacon, pancetta or chorizo
Optional but delicious!
1 red onion, diced
1 red pepper, diced
1 small carrot (optional)
peeled and finely diced

1 celery stick (optional)
finely diced
fresh garlic chopped, to taste
cube of beef or lamb stock
or vegetable stock cube
Mediterranean herbs
400g tin of chopped tomatoes
salt and pepper

Heat the olive oil in a large pan. Fry off the bacon or chorizo if using until browning. Add the chopped onion and fry until just browning. Add the mince and brown. Add the red pepper and fry. Add the carrot and celery (if using), and the garlic. Add the tomatoes and herbs. Simmer low and slow with a lid on. You can do this in a slow cooker.

The longer you cook it the more tender the meat
*Season to taste when cooked. Tastes even better the next day
so multiply up the recipe and freeze for
emergency future meals.*

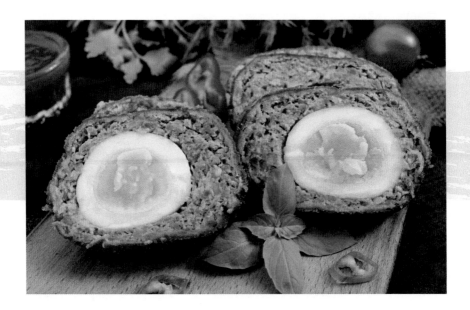

Scotch Eggs

6 peeled hard-boiled eggs
500g pork sausage meat
or pork mince
salt and pepper
2 tsp mustard

sage *or mixed herbs or other spices*
1 beaten egg
pork scratchings, *crushed*
Make your own or check packet that they are sugar free. Or you can use ground almonds.

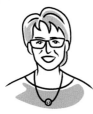

JEN

In a bowl, combine the sausage meat, seasoning, mustard and herbs and spices, mix well. I use my hands here. Divide the meat mixture into six and wrap each egg carefully.

Dip each in beaten egg and then the crushed cracklings. *This stage is a bit messy!*

Roast in a hot oven for 20 minutes.
Or until the pork is fully cooked, turning once during cooking.

A dish originally from England

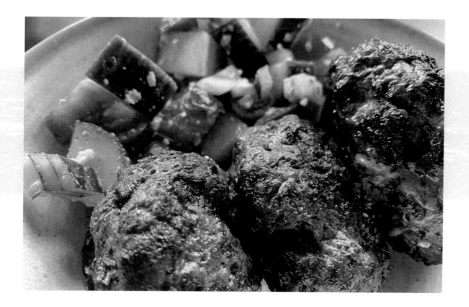

Dave's Kofte

2 lbs (1kg) ground beef (80/20)
½ bunch parsley, *finely chopped*
2 garlic cloves, *minced*

1 tbsp Aleppo pepper
zest of 1 lemon
salt and pepper *to taste*

Place the ground beef in a large mixing bowl. Combine the remaining ingredients. Add to ground beef and mix well to combine. **Cover and allow to chill for up to 24 hours.** I cook mine on the grill, but they can also be baked at 375° F for roughly 20 minutes

I could live on mince or ground meat, it is staple part of my diet. I prefer it over steak and you can't beat the price. You can do so much with it. One of my favourite ways to prepare it is sauté onion and bell pepper and set them aside, brown off 1000 g of ground beef (80/20). Keep breaking it up to form small pieces, add back in the onions and peppers.

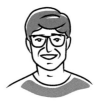

DAVE

Add chilli powder, paprika, cumin, salt and black pepper. Stir and finish with ½ cup of prepared sugar free salsa. A great one-pot, one-bowl meal.

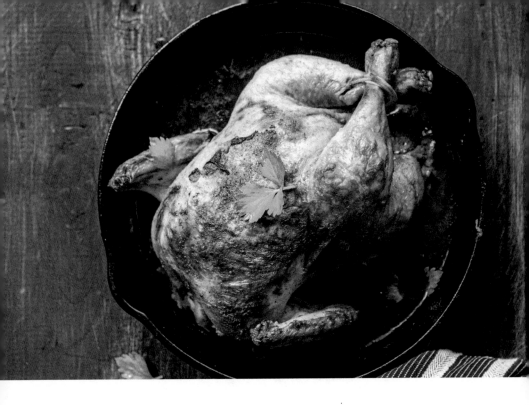

Chicken

*Versatile. Good for feeding a crowd.
I just roasted two large free-range chickens
because my daughter, son-in-law, and our four
grandchildren are coming around for tea.*

*Cover a chicken in fatty bacon and put half a lemon in the cavity to get a
nice moist chicken and a delicious lemony gravy in the bottom of the pan.
If you put the chicken in a large pot with a lid surrounded by celery, leek,
onion and green beans you also get everything cooked in one pot. This can
be done in a slow cooker. The leftovers make soup, too. I use thigh meat for
bakes and curries — it has an appealing texture and flavour.*

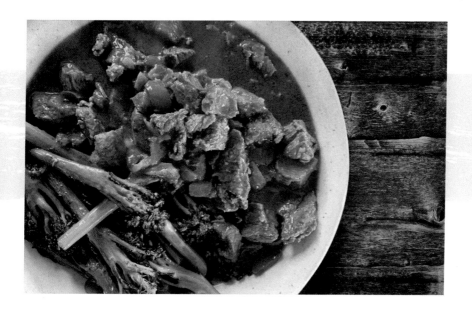

Chicken Butter Curry

A hit with us. My most frequently made recipe. Serve with green beans or cauliflower rice (page 96). You can also make it with lamb. Use your favourite spice mix or make your own. Have it as hot or mild as you like. Even more delicious on day two, so make plenty and have some for lunch at work or freeze the extra.

1 tbsp of ghee
or coconut oil for frying
1 tbsp of medium curry powder
Hot if you dare!
1 onion, chopped
1 red pepper, chopped
Salt and pepper

6 boneless, skinless chicken thighs
or 2 large chicken breasts, cubed
1 large tomato, chopped
or half a tin of chopped tomatoes
125g butter *or ghee*
ground almonds *to thicken (optional)*

Heat your saucepan and add a tablespoon of ghee or coconut oil. Add the curry powder and stir for a minute. Add the chopped onion and pepper. Stir and cook for about 3 minutes. Add the chicken, stir and cook for another few minutes. Add the chopped tomato and the butter or ghee. Stir. **Simmer gently for 20-30 minutes until cooked through.** Thicken the sauce with some ground almonds if needed.

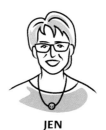

JEN

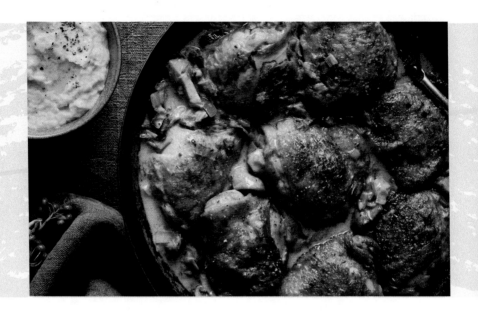

Chicken Thighs with Sage and Leek Cream Sauce

I have allowed 2 chicken thighs per person but depending on their size you may find one each is enough for some. In the photograph we have shown this with mashed swede (page 95) which is our favourite side to have with it or you could serve it with roasted veggies (page 97).

The dried porcini enrich the mushroom flavour and give an umami* hit to the recipe but you can omit them if you don't have them.

* Umami is the core fifth taste with sweet, sour, bitter, and salty. It means "essence of deliciousness" in Japanese and its taste is often described as the meaty, savory deliciousness that deepens flavor.

KATIE

Umami oh my!

SERVES 4

10g (¼oz) dried porcini mushrooms
8 medium chicken thighs, *skin on*
25g (1oz) butter
1 medium leek, *finely sliced*
250g (9oz) small chestnut
or button mushrooms, *halved*

16 broad sage leaves,
roughly chopped
150ml (5fl oz) dry white wine
100ml (3.5 fl oz) double cream
freshly ground black pepper
salt

Cover the porcini mushrooms with 50ml (2fl oz) warm water and leave to soak while you cook the chicken.

Fry the chicken thighs in a large, non-stick frying pan, skin-side down, for about 20 minutes or until rich golden brown. They will release fat from the skin as they cook. Season the chicken in the pan and turn when browned.

Cook for a further 15 minutes or so until golden brown. Transfer the chicken to a roasting tray and set aside.

If you have a lot of oil in the pan, tip some into a heatproof bowl to use another day, leaving a couple of tablespoons in the pan. **Add the butter to the pan and set over a medium-high heat.** When the butter is foaming, add the leek and mushrooms and stir-fry for about 15 minutes.

Drain the porcini mushrooms through a sieve and discard the water. Add these to the pan with the sage and stir through.

Add the chicken back into the pan, skin-side up.

Pour in the wine and bring to the boil. Reduce the wine for 5 minutes, then add the cream and once bubbling, reduce the heat to medium and let the chicken slowly bubble for about 20 minutes or until cooked through and falling off the bones. Serve straight away.

GET AHEAD
The chicken can be cooled and kept in the fridge for 3 days or frozen.
Defrost thoroughly before reheating to piping hot.

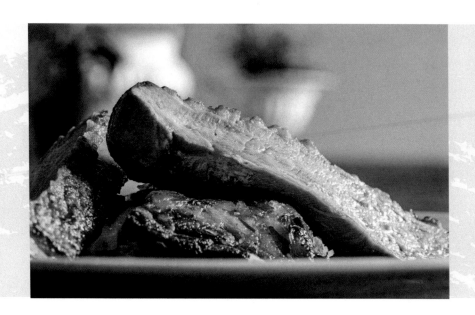

Duck

A healthy, fat-rich meal that's a succulent and satisfying addition to your menu.

Duck is darker in colour than chicken and turkey meats and is often cooked differently. By culinary standards, duck may be considered a red meat. Regardless of its classification as a white or red meat, duck is healthy, satisfying, and delicious.

Pick up duck eggs at the grocery or farmer's market
They're bigger than a chicken egg, cost a bit more, but have a special buttery flavour that's easy to love.

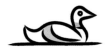

Georgia's Pan-Roasted Duck Breast with Crispy Skin

Sprinkle the skin of the duck breast with coarse salt and let the meat come to room temperature. If the skin is very thick, make very shallow cuts to the skin in a crosshatch pattern.

Pat the duck dry. Put 1 tablespoon of duck fat in a cold cast iron skillet, place the duck skin-side down in the skillet, and turn the heat on to medium-high.

As soon as the skin begins to crisp (5 minutes at most), turn heat down to medium-low. *If you like, you can cover the pan with a splatter guard that contains holes and allows air to circulate. (If you use a solid cover, the duck will steam and the skin will not stay crispy.)*

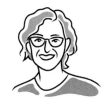

GEORGIA

Pour off excess fat as it renders to prevent burning.

Once the skin has cooked down to about half its original thickness (5–10 minutes, depending on how thick the skin is) and/or the internal temperature has reached about 125F (51C), **flip the duck over**, turn the heat up a pinch, and finish cooking for just a few more minutes to desired doneness. (I like it medium, around at 145F/63C.)

Let rest a bit before serving to retain natural juices

Jen's Easy Peasy Crispy Duck

Take one whole duck. Rub salt and Chinese five spice into the skin.

Roast in a hot oven (200c) for 30 minutes then turn the heat down to 100c and cook for a further 4 hours.

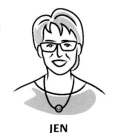

Remove from the oven and allow to rest for 15 minutes. The meat will be incredibly tender and the skin delicious!

JEN

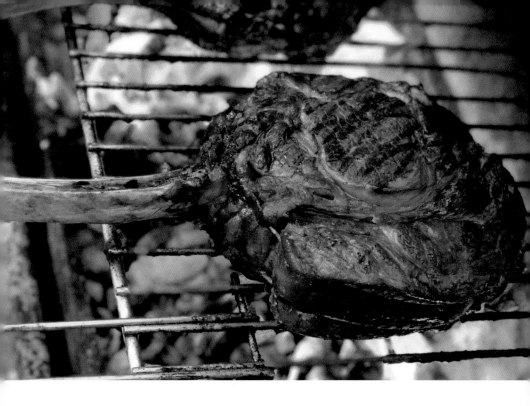

Beef

Cheap and versatile. Fatty minced beef is a versatile, nutrient dense choice. From good value mince up to indulgent filet steak and everything in between.

Cheap cuts like brisket, shin, or cheeks can be slow cooked to make their own delicious gravy. These are all favourites in our house. Served with red cabbage or celeriac mash. Real winter warmers. Ribeye is my favourite steak cut because it is fatty and still tender when cooked medium rare.
A big beef rib roast is a spectacular treat for a special occasion.
We often have one on Christmas Eve.

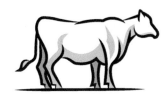

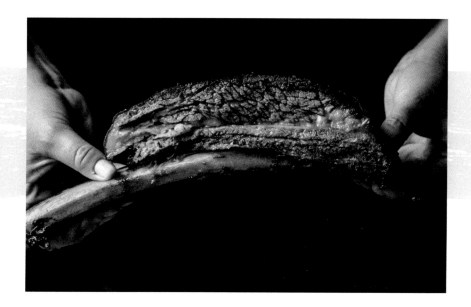

Short Ribs with Harissa and Olives

This recipe is a new invention born out of having some old olives in the fridge and half a jar of harissa that needed eating up! I've used the same recipe with shin beef (beef shank) and beef cheeks, all to good effect.

4 beef short ribs
from your local butcher
chopped chorizo *about 100g*
large red onion, *diced*
large red pepper, *diced*
3 tbsp olive oil

100g olives, *pitted*
garlic
4 large tomatoes, *quartered*
1 tbsp harissa paste
salt and pepper

Heat the oil in a large pan or casserole that has a lid. **Brown the meat on all sides**, add the onion and pepper and brown them. Add the chorizo, garlic, olives, tomatoes, harissa paste and some seasoning. Stir.

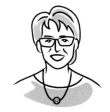

JEN

Put the lid on and cook in a low oven (100C) or in a slow cooker for about three hours or until the meat is coming off the bone. Adjust the seasoning.

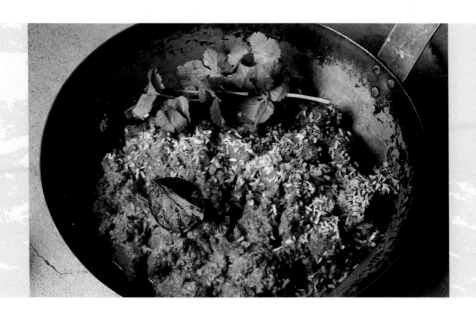

Malaysian Beef Rendang

Beef Rendang is a traditional Malaysian dish bursting with flavour from cardamon, star anise and lemongrass with natural sweetness from the coconut.

We learned this dish about 15 years ago from chef and friend Caroline Milli Artiss and have been making it ever since with a few twists of our own. You can use a muslin bag for the spices or pick them out as you see them. The curry lasts well so I often double the quantities. It is lovely with cauli rice.

KATIE

SERVES 6

FOR THE SPICE PASTE

75g (2½oz) piece of fresh ginger, *peeled*
fresh hot chillies or 1 teaspoon chilli flakes
1 medium onion, *quartered*

4 fat garlic cloves
2 lemongrass stalks,
outer layer removed

FOR THE CURRY

75g (2½oz) desiccated coconut
2 tbsp coconut
or extra virgin olive oil
6 cloves
8 cardamom pods
5 star anise
2 small cinnamon sticks
1kg (2lb 4oz) beef
(topside or stewing steak is fine) *cubed*

1 tbsp tamarind paste
or juice of ½ lemon
1 lemongrass stalk,
crushed at the end
4 lime leaves
400ml (14fl oz) coconut milk
2 tbsp tamari or
dark gluten-free soy sauce
coriander leaves, *to serve*

Dry-fry the coconut in a pan, stirring constantly until it turns brown and smells fantastic. Leave in a bowl to cool for later.

Put all the spice paste ingredients in a blender and with 2 tablespoons of water and blitz until it turns into paste.

Heat the oil in a large saucepan and add the spice paste, cloves, cardamom, star anise and cinnamon sticks and gently fry for about 5 minutes. Add the beef, tamarind, crushed lemongrass and lime leaves and fry until the beef turns brown, then add the coconut milk. Bring to the boil and then reduce the heat to its lowest setting and cover the pan.

Cook for 1 hour, checking every now and then to make sure there is still some liquid and it is not sticking to the bottom of the pan. If it starts to look dry, add a little water.

After an hour, remove the lid and leave to simmer for a further 30 minutes. This is meant to be a dry dish so this will let the liquid evaporate a little. When the beef is tender and falling apart it is ready, then add the toasted coconut (reserving a tablespoon to serve) and soy sauce and stir together. Taste and adjust the seasoning with salt if necessary. Serve straight away with the cauli rice.

GET AHEAD
*Cool the curry to room temperature and store in the fridge
for up to 5 days or freeze for up to 3 months.*

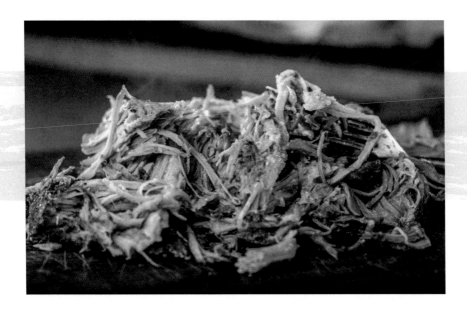

Trigger-Free Beef Barbacoa

1 large boneless beef chuck (*brisket*)
in 6 large cubes
1 beef stock cube
3 tsp dark chili powder
1 tbsp paprika
1 tbsp cayenne pepper

1 tbsp cumin powder
1 tbsp coriander
1 tbsp oregano
2 tbsp sea salt (*coarse*)
1 tbsp black pepper

Combine the spices. Cube the meat. Toss in spice mix.
Chill (if preparing the night before).
Sear. Dump in Crock Pot.
Add 1 cup Stock. Add 1 chili pepper (*optional*)

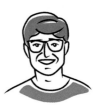

DAVE

Cook on low roughly 8 hours in a crock pot (slow cooker)
or low oven (100C, 200F)
Shred and enjoy. Serve with a bit of the meat sauce.

Add a chipotle pepper. Or two!

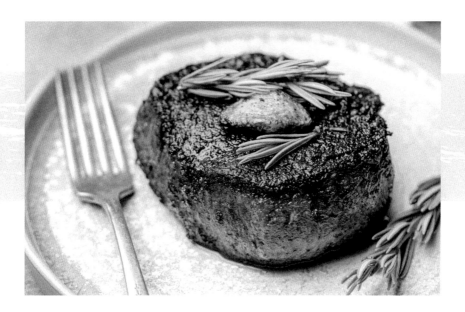

Perfectly Grilled Steak

Remove the steaks from the refrigerator and let sit, covered, at room temperature for about 20 minutes. Brush the steaks on both sides with olive oil and, this is important, *season generously with salt and pepper*.

Heat your grill to high about 5 minutes before grilling.

Cook until slightly charred for about 4-5 minutes. Poke with finger test to gauge doneness. Turn the steaks over and grill for 3-5 minutes for medium-rare, 5-7 minutes for medium, or 8-10 minutes for medium-well. Only turn once.

THE FINGER DONENESS TEST

| Raw | Rare | Medium Rare | Medium | Well Done |

Place on a cutting board and let rest 5 minutes before slicing.
Cut too early and your juices will escape.

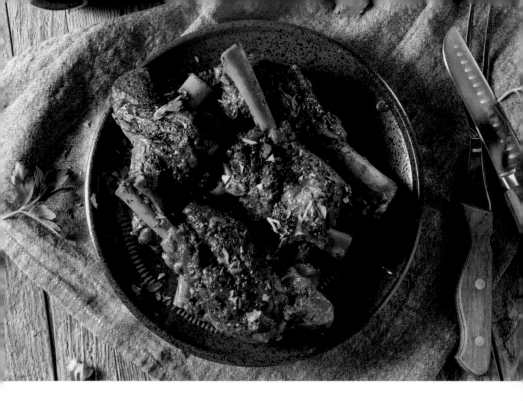

Lamb

Lamb is a wonderful meat.
Sheep are always raised on grass and the nutrition
profile is very good. Buy animals raised locally.
Befriending your local butcher
is a very good idea.

Lamb roasts are a treat. I make holes in my lamb leg or shoulder joints
and poke rosemary stalks and slithers of garlic into the skin. Give roasts a
30-minute sizzle in a hot oven and then turn the temperature down to finish
the cooking. I flash fry some lamb's liver every now and again. Delicious.
Slow cooking is also ideal with lamb and makes cooking so easy.

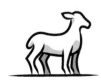

Slow-Cooked Lamb Shanks

Increase the amounts to make it for a family Sunday lunch. It's also a good idea to make extra portions of meals like this and put them in containers in the fridge or freezer for days when you have no meal prep time and need a speedy, satisfying hot meal. You can change the flavouring to curry or Moroccan spices. I add some chopped tomato if I do that.

I buy lamb shanks regularly from my local butcher. I love slow cooking as I can get my meal prep done and have a hot dinner ready at the end of the day. The shanks can also be served with green beans, roasted cauliflower, celeriac mash or red cabbage. Another alternative is to make the celeriac into 'roasties' or oven chips.

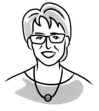

JEN

INGREDIENTS FOR TWO PEOPLE

1 tbsp fat *for frying*
ghee, tallow, lard or olive oil
2 lamb shanks
1 small onion, *chopped*

1 spring of rosemary
2 cloves of garlic *chopped*
salt and pepper

Heat a casserole dish or pan on your hob that has a lid and is large enough for the meat. Add a tablespoon of oil. Brown the shanks all over and then add the chopped onion, garlic, rosemary, salt and pepper.

Put the lid on and leave to cook on a gentle heat for about 10 minutes. Transfer to a low oven (100 degrees centigrade) and leave for at least two hours.

The meat should be falling off the bone. If not quite done allow another 30 minutes. Season to taste.

A warming and hearty meal for a cold day

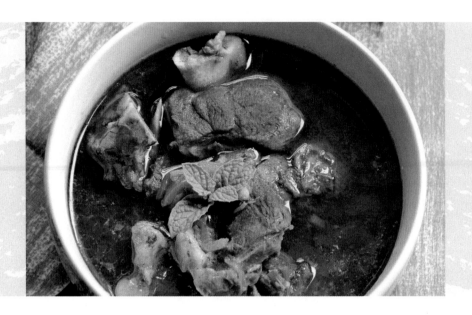

Giancarlo's Lamb One-Pot Supper

This rich and unctuous casserole is perfect for a family supper. The addition of low-carb swede (rutabaga) adds natural sweetness and helps to thicken the sauce.

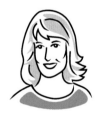

KATIE

Swede is a cross between turnips and cabbage

The taste is a milder than a turnip's when raw, and buttery and sweet-savory, though still a bit bitter, when cooked. They taste like Yukon Gold potatoes with flair. Swede has many national and regional names.

Swede is known as Rutabaga in North America

*From the Swedish word **rotabagge, rot (root) + bagge (lump, bunch).** In the U.S., the plant is also known as Swedish turnip or yellow turnip.*

SERVES 6

1.2 kilo stewing lamb
Diced into 4cm pieces
5 tbsp extra-virgin olive oil
2 tsp salt
freshly-ground black pepper
50g butter
1 onion, *thickly sliced*
2 cloves garlic
peeled and lightly crushed

1 sprig of rosemary
350g swede (*rutabaga*)
Cut into 2cm cubes
200g chestnut mushrooms
200ml white wine or stock
3 tbsp tomato puree
250g baby spinach leaves

Put the lamb with the oil in a shallow pan over a medium heat. Allow the water from it to evaporate for around 10 minutes or until it browns all over. Use a slotted spoon to transfer the lamb to a bowl leaving the oil in the pan.

Now add the butter to the pan and fry the vegetables, garlic and rosemary for 5 to 7 minutes until lightly browned.

Add the lamb back into the pan and pour in the wine. Bring it to the boil and reduce for five minutes before adding the tomato paste and 300ml hot water. Stir through and reduce the heat to simmer.

Cover the casserole and let it cook for 1.5 hours or until the meat is tender and falls apart easily. Add a little more water as necessary if it starts to dry.

When you are just ready to eat,
stir in the spinach leaves and replace the lid.
Cook for a few minutes until they have wilted. Then serve.

Low carb yet naturally sweet

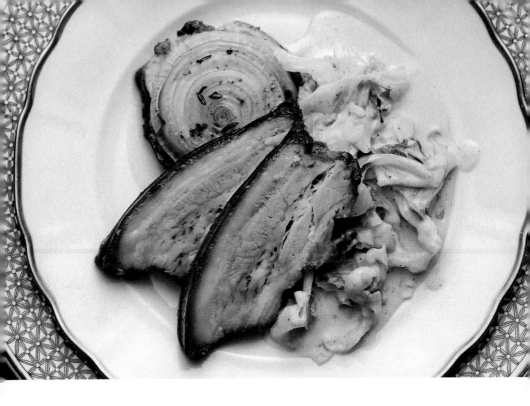

Pork

*Thanks to our friends at DietDoctor.com
for this lovely, nutritious pork dish.*

*If you don't have pointed cabbage, regular cabbage is fine! You can prepare
the cabbage ahead of time and just warm and serve when the meat is done.
It's a perfect way to enjoy your guests instead of focusing on the meal.
The apple does have some sugar in it, and onions contain some carbs.
To make this dish more strictly keto, just leave the apples
and onions in the pan after roasting the pork.*

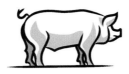

Roasted Pork Belly with Creamed Pointed Cabbage

2½ lbs (1.1kg) pork belly
2 tbsp sea salt
1 tbsp fennel seeds
½ tsp ground black pepper
½ tsp cloves
1 tbsp olive oil
1 (4 oz.) yellow onion
1 apple *(optional)*

CREAMED CABBAGE
2 lbs pointed cabbages
1 tbsp butter
¼ cup heavy whipping cream
¼ cup cream cheese
salt and pepper

Preheat the oven to 350°F (175°C).
Dry the pork with a paper towel. The skin should be very dry.

Using a sharp knife, score the skin and fat but be careful not to cut the meat.
Grind spices and mix with salt. Rub mixture all around the pork belly, making an
effort to get some of the rub into each score. Drizzle olive oil on top and rub in.

Place the meat skin side down in a greased baking dish. Bake on a lower rack
for about two hours, depending on thickness. Use a thermometer and let the
internal temperature reach 180°F (80°C) before you remove the pork from the
oven. While the pork is baking, slice onion and optional apple.

Lift up the meat and place on a clean dish. Put the sliced onion and apple in the
middle of the baking dish. Place the meat on top with the skin side up.

Increase the oven temperature to 400°F (200°C) and place the dish back in the
oven for 30 minutes or until the skin is golden brown and crispy. Let the meat
rest for a couple of minutes before you slice and serve it.

While the meat is baking, prepare the cabbage.
Divide lengthwise and remove the core. Slice coarsely.

Fry the cabbage over medium heat in butter until soft but not brown.
Season with salt and pepper to taste. Add cream and cream cheese and stir.
Lower the heat and let simmer until the cream is slightly thickened.

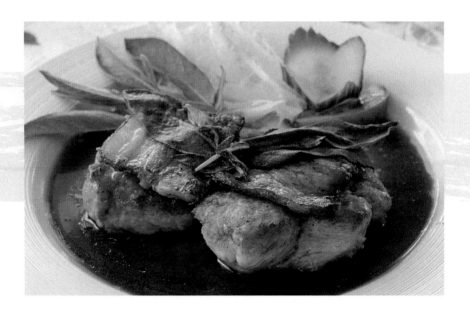

Saltimbocca

2 lbs (1kg) pork loin
cut into 8 equal sections
8 slices prosciutto
8 sage leaves
2 tbsp olive oil

2 tbsp butter
juice of 1 lemon
½ glass white wine *(optional)*
2 tbsp capers *(optional)*
2 cloves of garlic

ANNA

Place a piece of pork in a large storage bag and pound flat. Repeat for each cutlet. (You can find pork cutlets at most stores if you prefer a short cut.)

Lay each piece of prosciutto flat, and place a sage leaf on the top, centre of each piece. Place a cutlet on top of each piece of prosciutto and wrap each cutlet. Add olive oil to a large skillet and heat to medium high. Add cutlets and cook for about 2- 3 minutes per side.

Remove cutlets from the pan, and place on a platter. Add lemon juice and wine, reduce by half. Add garlic and butter. Whisk together. Add cutlets back to the pan, and sauté on each side for about 1 -2 minutes. Add capers, and serve.

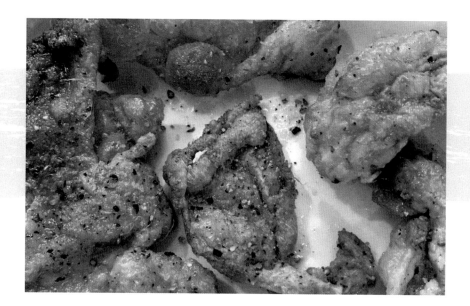

Pork Scratchings

I know we shouldn't be snacking, but sometimes I just want something after my meal. These are also good for making a crunchy coating on scotch eggs or chicken goujons. If I'm going to a party, I take some as they always go over well and give me something to eat!

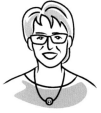

JEN

Ask your butcher for pork skin with the fat on
Get them to chop it up for you into cubes

Place the cubes on a large roasting tray, spread out. Roast on a high heat for about 15-20 minutes until the cubes are browned and crackled but not burned. Remove from the fat and add salt. Save the fat for cooking.

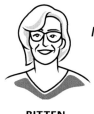

My favourite meal is Swedish thick "bacon"
(pork belly) with mashed cauliflower, butter, and a sprinkle of nutmeg.

BITTEN

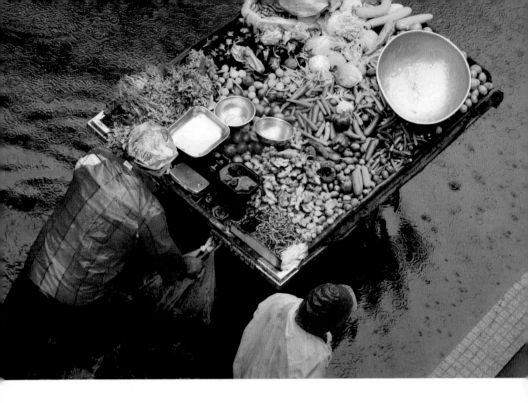

Vegetables

Vegetables and side dishes are good to add interest and volume to a meal. How much you have them is up to you and your preferences.

Some meals I have quite a bit of veg and some days I just eat meat and fat. I tried the carnivore diet but it got a bit boring for me long-term. Cauliflower is really versatile. I find it delicious roasted. You can melt some ghee and toss your cauliflower florets in it, season and roast for about 15-20 minutes. You can also do the same with a whole cauliflower (this takes longer obviously but makes a good centrepiece) or cauliflower steaks, add your favourite herbs and spices. You can roast or boil cauliflower and then mash or puree with a blender to make cauliflower mash. Add garlic and butter for even more deliciousness. One of my favourite uses of cauliflower is to make a rice substitute.

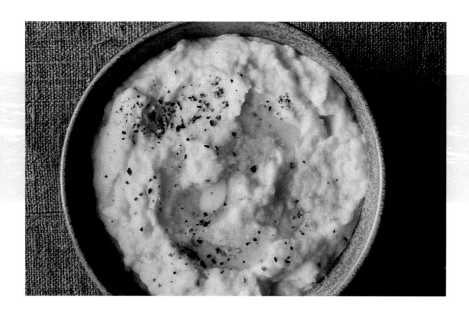

Mashed Swede

This pale orange mash is delicately spicy and slightly sweet. It makes a creamy contrast to any main course and any leftovers are wonderful with bacon and eggs.

SERVES 6

400g (14oz) swede
*diced roughly into
about 3cm (1¼in) cubes*
50g (1¾oz) butter

100ml (3½fl oz) double cream
½ teaspoon nutmeg *(optional)*
salt and freshly ground black pepper

Boil the swede in salted water for 25–30 minutes until tender.
Drain the swede through a colander and put it into a food processor to blend or back into the pan and use a potato masher.

Add the remaining ingredients and blend again until smooth. Taste and adjust the seasoning as necessary.

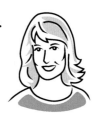

KATIE

Serve straight away.
Or put into a serving dish and keep warm.

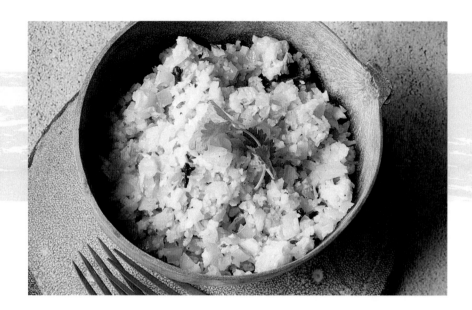

Cauliflower Rice

1 large cauliflower
olive oil, *coconut oil or ghee*
herbs, *spices optional to taste*

This is the messy bit! Cut your cauliflower into chunks. No
need to remove all the stork and leaves as you can use these
bits. Whizz up the chunks in 30 second blasts in a food
processor. Or you can use a cheese grater if you don't have
a blender. There are three ways to cook your rice. In the
microwave for 3 minutes, fried up with olive oil or ghee for
5-10 minutes (you may need a little liquid and can add in spring
onions) or roasted, again with oil.

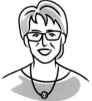

JEN

Experiment with what you like best

*Cauli rice goes really well with the chicken curry. You can also use the raw
rice cold in a salad like a fake couscous, just add olive oil, lemon juice,
spring onion, chopped tomato and fresh herbs and seasoning.*

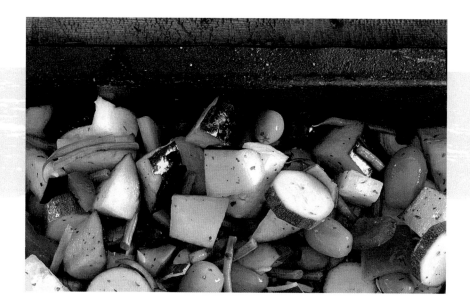

Roast Mediterranean Vegetables

This goes great with lamb, beef roasts, chicken, and meatballs.

1 large red onion	2 courgettes *(zucchini)*
1 large red pepper	4 tbsp olive oil
1 large aubergine *(eggplant)*	Mediterranean herbs
cherry tomatoes *small punnet*	salt and pepper

Chop all the vegetables in to chunks and place in a large roasting tray.
Add the oil and seasoning and mix.

Bake in a hot oven for about 30 minutes. Stir halfway through.

Celeriac (celery root) is a useful vegetable
Quite a chore to peel but makes a great mash to go with stews.
Can also be cut into chunks for chips or roasting. Treat it like potato.
If you can eat cream, it makes a wonderful dauphinoise.

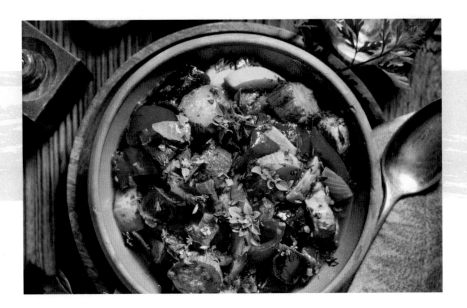

Ratatouille

A similar idea to the Roast Mediterranean vegetables on page 97, but this recipe has a more sauce-like quality.

1 large red onion
1 large red pepper
1 large aubergine (eggplant)
2 courgettes (zucchini)
fresh garlic *to taste*

500g of passata
(uncooked tomato puree)
or chopped tomatoes
4 tbsp olive oil
Mediterranean herbs
salt and pepper

Chop all the vegetables. Fry the onion and pepper in the olive oil. Add the chopped aubergine, courgette and garlic. Stir. Add the tomato and seasoning. Simmer for 30 minutes or so until everything is cooked down.

Flavour improves the next day. Make plenty!

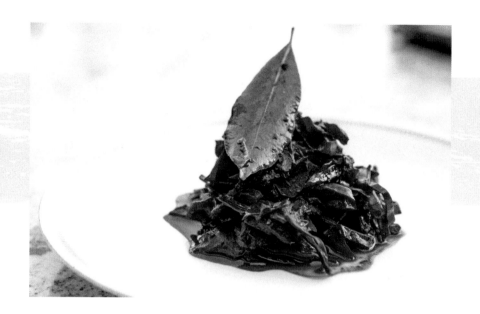

Red Cabbage

White cabbage fried in butter is a quick, delicious dish and goes wonderfully with Bolognese (do it as ribbons) or stew. Red cabbage takes a bit more cooking but is worth the effort occasionally and especially in the winter with slow cooked casseroles. Traditional recipes have sugar in but it works really well without.

1 red cabbage, *chopped*
1 red onion, *chopped*
2 tbsp olive oil *or ghee*

2 tbsp balsamic *or red wine vinegar*
small glass of water *or stock*
salt and pepper

Fry the red onion in the oil until just browning, add the cabbage and stir fry for a few minutes. Add the vinegar and liquid, put a lid on and simmer gently for about 30 minutes, stirring occasionally. Season. Keeps for a couple of days in the fridge and can be microwaved to re-heat.

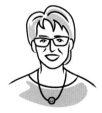

JEN

More Vitamin C than oranges

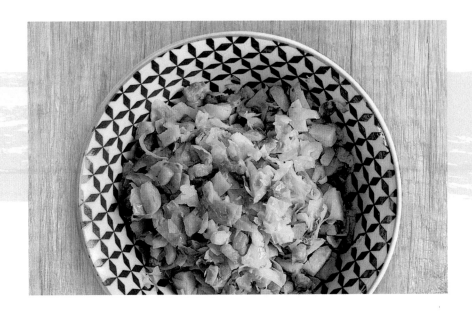

Stir-Fried Sprouts with Pancetta

We have this on Christmas day with our turkey but there's no reason not to have it on other days!

200g small Brussels sprouts
100g chopped pancetta *or bacon*
pine nuts *(optional)*
2 tbsp olive oil

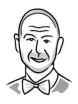

DAVID

Chop the sprouts into quarters.
Fry the pancetta in a hot pan with the oil until browning.
Add the pine nuts if using and fry for another minute.
Add the sprouts and keep frying and stirring for about
5-10 minutes until browning and cooked through.

Enjoy on Holidays — and Tuesdays

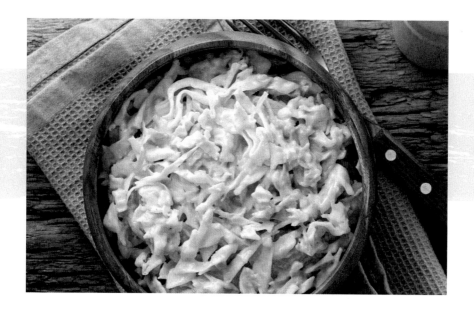

Coleslaw

Perfect with cold fish or meats and good for buffets.

1 medium white cabbage
1 small red onion
or bunch of spring onion
2 large carrots

2 tsp mustard
2 tbsp mayonnaise
1 tbsp Balsamic *or white wine vinegar*
salt and pepper

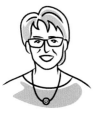

JEN

Grate/shred the cabbage, onion and carrot
in a food processor or by hand.

In a large bowl combine with the rest of the ingredients.
I sometimes add some mixed seeds for a bit of crunch.

Perfect for picnicking!

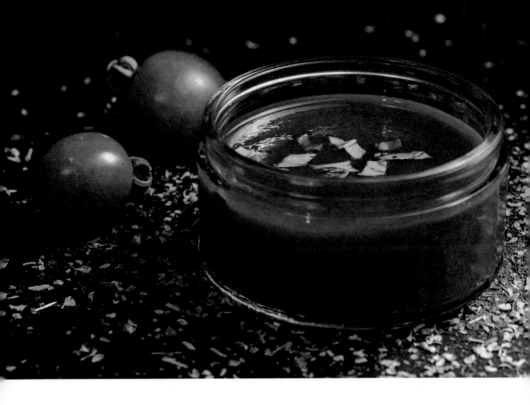

Sauces

My mother-in-law can't stand a dry dinner and I tend to agree with her. Sauces can definitely make a meal.

We need to be cautious because often the reason that sauces are delicious is that they have sugar. Here are some safe versions that don't disappoint flavourwise.

Make your own ketchup
Use tomato paste, water, white vinegar — or use apple cider vinegar as a base. Then add seasonings until you get the flavour you like: sea salt, onion powder, garlic powder, paprika, ground cloves, and mustard powder.

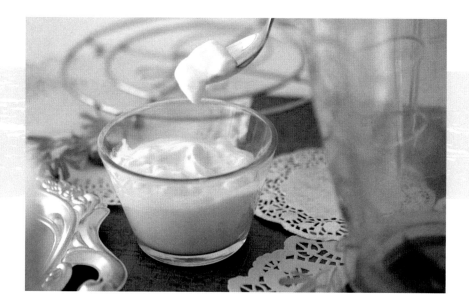

Mayonnaise

There are some shop-bought mayonnaises that are sugar free but they are hard to locate and mostly still have poor quality fats in them. It is ridiculously easy to make your own if you have a hand blender and the tall pot it came with.

1 egg
250ml liquid oil
(Melted ghee or bacon fat, or light olive oil or MCT oil)

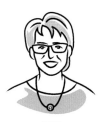

Crack the egg and gently lower it into the pot. Carefully poor the oil over the egg. Place your blender over the egg yolk right at the bottom of the pot.

. JEN

Blend starting at the bottom and slowly lifting the blender out as you go.

Make lots of variations

Add mustard, garlic, lemon zest, fresh herbs, or curry paste.

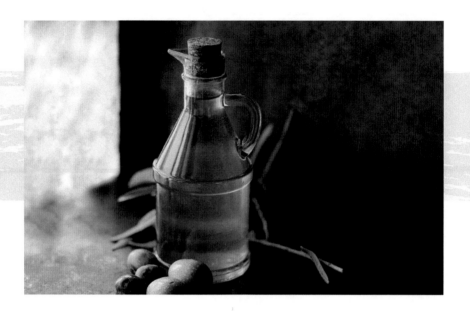

Salad Dressing

Many shop-bought dressings have added sugar or poor-quality oils.
It's easy to make your own and keep it in a jar in the fridge.

200ml avocado
or olive oil
1 tsp mustard

50ml balsamic
or white wine vinegar or lemon juice
salt and pepper

Put everything in a jar with a lid and shake until combined.

Add spices, herbs or garlic

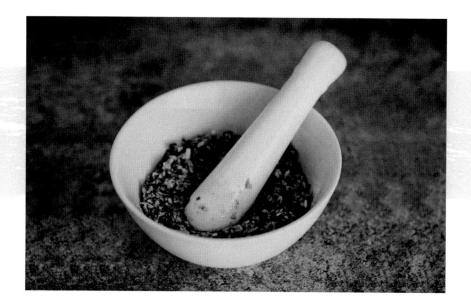

Pesto

This goes beautifully with fish, lamb, steak or on salads. Traditionally made with parmesan and pine nuts too. I now make this simpler version which is still delicious but do add parmesan and pine nuts if you are okay with them. Keeps really well in the fridge.

1 large bunch basil
300ml olive oil

garlic cloves *to taste*
salt and pepper

Take the basil leaves off their stalks and put everything in a big jug. Blend.

A summer favourite

JEN

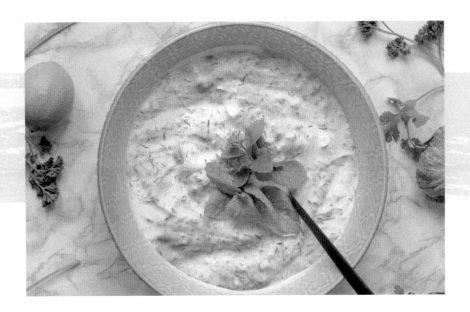

Herb and Yoghurt Sauce

This goes really well with salmon and asparagus or green beans. I don't have it much now since being really careful with dairy but I've included it as it's so simple and delicious.

50g mixed fresh herbs	2 tbsp lemon juice
— *mint, dill, chives, parsley*	salt and pepper
4 tbsp olive oil	300g full-fat Greek yoghurt

Whizz everything together in a food processor or with your hand blender. Keeps for 4 days in the fridge.

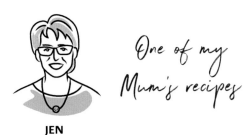

One of my
Mum's recipes

JEN

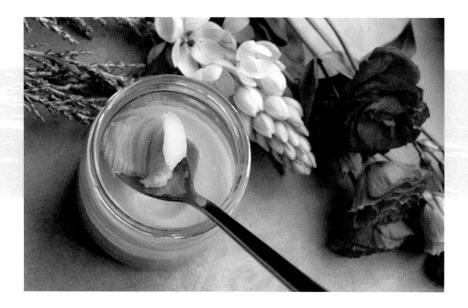

Ghee

You can buy ghee but it's often expensive. It's much easier to make your own as you need it. The advantage of ghee is that it can be used for high heat cooking because the proteins from the butter have been removed. It's also therefore suitable for people with lactose intolerance and sugar addicts. It has a lovely flavour.

3 packs of unsalted butter *Get grass fed if you can afford it*

Place in a large pan over a slow heat and bring to a gentle simmer.
Simmer for about 15 minutes and you will see the froth rise to the top.
Skim this off carefully and keep going until its nearly clear. Strain your ghee into clean jars using a very fine sieve or muslin. Can also be made in a Crock Pot or slow cooker.

Use as cooking fat.
Makes lovely fried eggs

DAVID

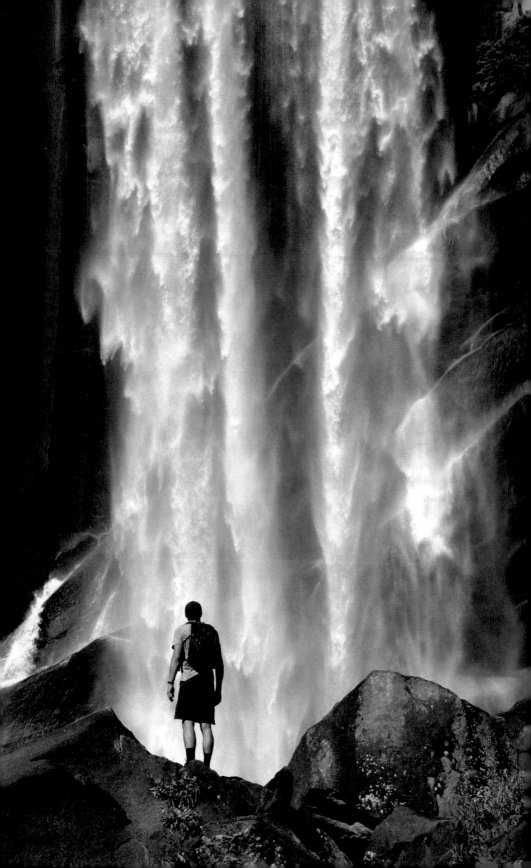

CHAPTER 5

Healing Your Addicted Brain

The structure and function of your brain is altered by eating sugar and refined carbohydrates.

Like other addictive substances, sugar has a physical effect on the body and the brain.

This is definitely something I wish I had known when I was younger. Also, I hope this information makes us all think more than twice about giving sugary treats to children as rewards and entertainment. We wouldn't give them alcohol or drugs, after all.

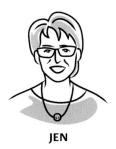

JEN

The food we eat is very important for carbohydrate addicts in recovery but it is only part of the whole long-term recovery process. I talked in Chapter 1 about how sugar and refined foods can hijack important processes in the body and brain. Every biological system operates with complex feedback mechanisms in an effort to maintain balance. Nature is very clever. If we eat too much sugar, along with insulin, we get high dopamine and serotonin which makes us feel good temporarily.

Over the long term though, the brain down-regulates these raised neurotransmitters by reducing the number of receptors. We need more and more carbs just to feel okay. When we rely on sugar and junk food to feel good it is like going down a rabbit hole, constantly trying to bolster ourselves with what we eat but never getting to a place of wellbeing. So, when we finally decide we must crawl back out of the hole, it's essential to find new and better ways of feeling good and balancing neurotransmitters for wellbeing. Otherwise, we are much more likely to succumb to the inevitable cravings and temptations all around us and lose hope of getting free.

Dopamine, oxytocin, serotonin and endorphins play important roles in our sense of well-being and brain health. I'll explain the function of each of these and how to get your daily DOSE of each one so that you are fighting fit for your recovery journey.

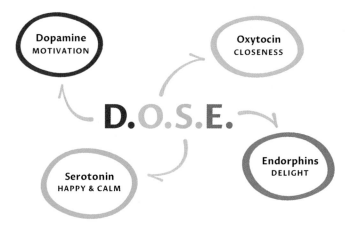

Dopamine

Dopamine is involved in reward and motivation. It sends signals to other nerve cells. Just the anticipation of a reward (such as carbs) increases dopamine in the brain. Many addictive drugs act by increasing the availability of dopamine in the brain. Dopamine is also involved in movement. Parkinson's disease is a lack of dopamine, for example. Dopamine signals for us to repeat 'desirable' behaviours such as eating carby foods. High levels of dopamine are also implicated in impulsive behaviour. For example, in food addiction it's likely that the dopamine released in response to food cues (seeing, smelling or even thinking about food) makes it difficult for us to stop the action of reaching for that food. I have experienced this phenomenon myself repeatedly. I would 'decide' not to eat sugar but then watch my hand reaching for a biscuit when I saw the packet. It felt like aliens had taken over my brain! I just couldn't understand how in other life situations I could have such self-control, but never with food. We are powerfully driven by our brain chemistry.

Another action of dopamine is that when a certain behaviour, such as eating, leads to dopamine release, the brain is altered in a way that makes that behaviour more easily triggered in the future.

Nicotine is another drug that increases dopamine leading to addiction over time. Cravings for specific foods can persist long after you have stopped eating them because of this re-wiring of the brain. Cravings are triggered by situational stimuli linked to the eating behaviour in the past such as smells, sights, locations or people. Even now I get these cravings but they are lesser and easier to resist as I develop new associations and habits. Psychological and neurological recovery takes many times longer than the physical withdrawal from using carbs as fuel.

Dopamine is also involved in pain processing and might be implicated in conditions like fibromyalgia. Lots of patients I have met have noticed improvement in chronic pain conditions after quitting table sugar and refined carbohydrates.

Carbs, caffeine and nicotine deliver short term dopamine highs but can underlie addictive behaviours by reducing dopamine in the long run and making those behaviours harder to resist.

Low levels of dopamine have been linked with apathy, fatigue, low mood, poor concentration and memory, all of which I suffered from at times. An important part of recovery is getting dopamine in balance.

How do we get our daily dopamine in natural, healthy ways?

1. **Dopamine is made from tyrosine or phenylalanine which is in protein rich foods like beef, pork, fish, chicken, cheese and seeds.** So, make sure you stick to the green foods list in Chapter 3 and base your meals on good quality protein.

2. **After nutrition, regular exercise is just about the brain's best medicine.** It increases new brain cells, helping you to re-wire your brain, slows down brain aging and increases dopamine. Find anything you enjoy that is active and notice how you feel before and after. David and I often joke that we never feel worse for exercise, no matter how little we wanted to do it in the first place. Make some new habits around physical activity being a daily priority. Walking, jogging, dancing, gardening, badminton, golf, yoga it doesn't matter, just get moving! Prolonged sitting will lower dopamine. Eating and weight gain has often robbed us of the motivation to move around. Don't think of exercise for weight loss or as punishment for eating but as the ultimate mood booster.

3. **Pay attention to stress levels.** Easier said than done sometimes but worth always keeping in mind and learning how to keep stress at the right level for you. Meditation, massage and yoga have all been shown to increase dopamine. Learn not to take on too much. Be good to yourself.

4. Make good sleep a priority. Go to bed and get up at regular times allowing for enough sleep. Turn screens off well before bedtime or invest in some blue light blocking glasses. Even one night's poor sleep can downregulate dopamine receptors. Research also shows that we are much more likely to over eat after a bad night. Talking of screens, beware social media and games on your phone. They too can get you trapped in a bad cycle. I had to delete a well-known game off my phone as I was spending way too much time on it.

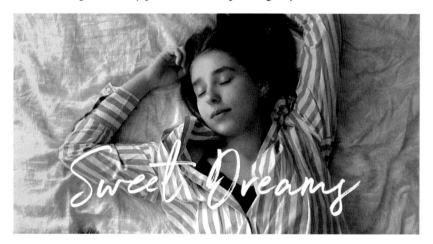

5. Listening to music seems to increase our dopamine levels. Get listening to your favourite music, or maybe playing!

6. Pick hobbies that provide new discoveries or challenges. This can be sporting, such as playing with a team, or trying to beat your personal best or it could be something like birdwatching or gardening where there are always new discoveries to be made. This mimics the survival role dopamine had for our ancestors in finding food sources and shelter. Try and develop a new skill or return to something you loved as a younger person. I'm a big knitter, which gives me something constructive and enjoyable to do in the evenings other than eating!

7. Celebrate small wins every day. Make a list of stuff to do and enjoy ticking things off. Savour small victories.

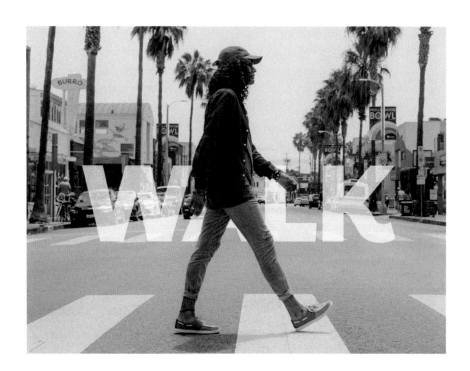

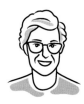 **ANNA** *I walk daily for 30-60 minutes, and I mean mosey. This kind of walking helps your body destress and burn fat efficiently. I also use the X3 Bar for muscle development. I use this for 10 minutes per day 6 days per week. Muscle is valuable real-estate, and I don't want to lose any.*

Interestingly, anyone can gain muscle despite age. Sarcopenia is the leading cause of frailty in seniors. I prioritize my muscle building for that reason, as well as a host of others. Bone density preservation, youthful skin, strength, and a healthy metabolism.

Over the past year I have put on 10 pounds without going up at all in size. This tells me I lost fat and gained muscle. Yay! That was what I wanted. More youthful, metabolically active muscle.

Oxytocin

Oxytocin is a hormone released in the brain which is most commonly linked with bonding, reproduction and childbirth. There have also been suggestions that it plays a role in suppressing appetite. Higher oxytocin is linked to lower susceptibility to substance use disorders. Also, oxytocin seems to inhibit fear and produce antidepressant and anti-inflammatory effects in animals. Oxytocin is essentially the hormone of closeness. It might be that for some of us, we have replaced closeness to others with the process of eating over time. Evolutionarily, eating and closeness were inextricably linked, we shared food to survive. Certainly, in some families food is a substitute for emotional closeness.

What are some natural ways to boost oxytocin?

1. **Yoga and meditation boost oxytocin.**

2. **Listening to or participating in music** boots oxytocin.

3. **Giving or receiving a massage** have been shown to raise oxytocin levels.

4. **Sharing time and feelings with friends and loved ones** increases wellbeing and closeness.

5. **There is some evidence that sharing food and eating itself increases oxytocin.** Make sure you still eat meals with others whilst sticking to your food plan. I absolutely love to cook big family meals and cater for a crowd. I just make stuff I want to eat like big stews and roasts with delicious sides. Everyone is happy to join in!

6. **Physical closeness such as holding hands and hugging with partners and friends can trigger oxytocin production** and don't forget to give the dog or cat a good stroke!

7. **Both the skin and the stomach like warmth for comfort.** Relaxing in the bath or steam room or sitting in the sun can be relaxing and oxytocin boosting. Hot soup on a winter's day makes us feel cosy and safe.

Add closeness and comfort in your life

Serotonin

Serotonin is a vital chemical made by nerves in the body. It is actually mostly produced in the gut. So, we do have 'gut feelings'! Serotonin plays a central role in keeping us happy, calm and focused. Some anti-depressant medications (like Prozac for instance) work by increasing the amount of serotonin available in the brain. Low levels can lead to irritability, poor attention and low mood. Also, it's worth noting again that high sugar and carbohydrate foods lead to a short-term boost in serotonin due to insulin allowing extra tryptophan into the brain. However, the down side is that repeated over time this leads to less available tryptophan and less serotonin. The brain also reduces serotonin receptors. So, although you get a short-term boost from your chocolate bar it's a very poor long-term strategy.

How can we boost the levels of this important feel-good stuff naturally? Fortunately, there are several strategies which all have good evidence to back them up, for you to incorporate in your daily life.

1. **Nutrition is important.** Make sure you get foods that contain trypto-phan, an amino acid from protein that is converted into serotonin in the body. Tryptophan rich foods are low in carbohydrate and include chicken, turkey, eggs, fish, cheese, pumpkin seeds and sesame seeds. Although increasing dietary tryptophan doesn't appear to directly boost serotonin, it makes sense to have plenty available.

2. **Exercise can help.** Aerobic exercises such as brisk walking, jogging, dancing or cycling have been shown to increase serotonin. Human beings evolved to move. Yet again, our modern way of life doesn't fit with our basic biology. It's really important to find an activity that you enjoy and do regularly. Walking is absolutely fine. Yoga can also be helpful; several studies show it boots serotonin. You can further boost the beneficial effects of exercise on serotonin levels by doing it outdoors, especially in bright light. Light levels during the day are related to serotonin production. Not at night though, when you want serotonin converted into melatonin, the sleep hormone, so turn off screens and bright lights in the evening or invest in blue light blockers!

3. **Sunlight is important** for the body's production of vitamin D which promotes serotonin production. A good proportion of us suffer from the winter blues and need to make special efforts to eat well, exercise and get outdoors in the winter to maintain our wellbeing and in summer to boost our vitamin D stores. Personally, I take a vitamin D supplement between October and March.

4. **Happy memories and pleasant thoughts directly lead to serotonin release.** How about keeping a special file of photos on your phone with your happiest moments? You could even set it to your favourite music and play it a couple of times a day for a natural boost! There is plenty of evidence that reviewing your day for things that went well and you are grateful for can boost mood over time. Try and develop this habit at bedtime. It's easy to fall into the trap of worrying about things and focusing on our supposed flaws. Human beings survived by being sensitive to 'threat' information. We can re-train ourselves to notice things that have gone well and that we can feel good about.

GEORGIA *I like to vary my exercise depending on the weather and season so I don't get bored: 10-mile bike rides, half-hour hikes in the hills, vigorous 3-mile walks with hand weights around my local reservoir (or other car-free path), 3-mile jogs, snowshoeing at night (no lights needed!), 30-minute strength training routines to dance music, mini-trampoline workouts, even raking leaves or shovelling snow.*

Serotonin gives us feelings of happiness and well-being

Endorphins

Endorphins are 'endogenous morphine' like substances. That means they are molecules produced inside the body that reduce pain perception and produce feelings of euphoria. Endorphins are needed when we are injured or stressed but can also be released by eating delicious food, listening to music, taking vigorous exercise or laughing! How can we get more of these natural pain killers and mood boosters?

1. **Yet again, exercise is high on the list!** Everyone has heard of the runner's high. Research suggests that you need to exercise for at least 30 minutes to get the endorphin boost. Moderate intensity seems best. There is some evidence that group exercise works even better than solo for this effect.

2. **Meditation is another way to trigger endorphins,** try one of the apps in the resources chapter or sign up for a local yoga or meditation class.

3. **Laughter is the best medicine.** Try watching a half hour comedy with friends or family. People shown comedy shows post-operatively have been shown to experience less pain and anxiety.

4. **Random acts of kindness** for other people trigger endorphin release, maybe make this a regular habit in some way. Donate to the food bank or pay forward a coffee next time you get one. Volunteer for a local good cause. I volunteer as a local walk leader once a week, combining exercise, fresh air and socialising!

5. **Music can definitely boost mood,** performing music seems to particularly boost endorphins. Singing in choirs has been shown to improve wellbeing.

6. **Spicy food is thought to trigger endorphin release** so try the curry recipe on page 75 in Chapter 4 with a few extra chillies!

Dance to your favourite song to release endorphins

In dealing with any addiction the necessary removal of the substance can bring about a sense of loss. I hope these ideas help you to choose some new more adaptive habits to cultivate.

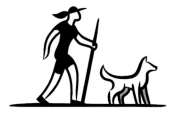

Prioritise exercise. It has benefits for mental and physical wellbeing across the board

Choose something you enjoy and can do regularly. I find it really helps to think of how we evolved. Both in terms of the food environment but also how we lived day to day as cave man and woman. There would have been plenty of movement and plenty of communication about shared priorities. We would have been outside most of the day in all weathers. Activities like walking, gardening, rearing animals, caring for children and older people, singing, cooking and making things feel 'primal' and for that reason are good for our wellbeing. What would your role have been in the tribe? Maybe do more of that! See what feels right to you.

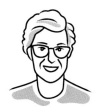

ANNA *I take things one day at a time. It's the only day I have! I "feed" what I want to grow, my relationships, my business, (which I consider my life's purpose), my health, my spirit, and my mind. I feed all these areas of my life with time, care, attention, love, affection, action, meditation, learning, and practicing a way of living that supports the vision I have for myself. A life of dignity, health, purpose, friendship, and integrity. I walk almost daily, attend and host regularly scheduled recovery meetings, work with others, have a sponsor I am in regular contact with, and practice gratitude.*

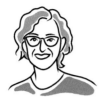 **GEORGIA** *Those of us who struggle with food and weight were taught to believe that we are in complete control over our appetite and eating behaviour—that if we simply commit to eating less and exercising more, we can easily reach and maintain a healthy weight for life. This overly simplistic conventional "wisdom" has repeatedly failed us because it ignores the powerful role that food quality, hormones, and neurotransmitters play in the sophisticated and carefully controlled system of appetite regulation. More than two dozen different brain and body chemicals are listening to the foods we eat... and changing our behaviour in response.*

As Dr Unwin has so beautifully described: if we eat the wrong foods, our brain chemistry can become seriously unbalanced, throwing our emotions and behaviours into turmoil.

Living creatures did not evolve to require calculators and calorie charts to know how much food to eat. *Metabolically healthy animals, including humans, naturally eat the right amount of food—they don't have to fight cravings, worry about unhealthy weight gain, or exercise to burn off excess calories. Simply put, they can trust their instincts. Our appetite "thermostats" evolved to regulate themselves without our having to think about it...so long as we eat a species-appropriate whole foods diet.*

But when we consume modern refined carbohydrates like sugar, flour, fruit juice, and cereal products every day, multiple times per day, from very early childhood forward, our blood sugar levels repeatedly spike to unnatural extremes, dragging insulin, stress hormones, appetite regulation hormones, and many other hormones along for the ride.

This invisible hormonal roller coaster can destabilize mood, energy, and concentration levels, causing anxiety and carbohydrate cravings to occur between meals.

Over time, this dangerous way of eating can damage our appetite thermostat, tricking us into thinking we need more food than we actually do. *When blood sugar and insulin levels are extremely unstable, it may feel as if our emotions are driving our desire to eat—yet what is actually happening is that our eating is driving our emotions.*

 *It only takes a matter of days to bring yourself to a safer and healthier place*

And it is well worth the effort—but for those of us who have become addicted to these foods, it can feel impossible to step off that roller coaster. Sadly, unlike most other addictions, sugar and other food addictions often begin in early childhood when our impressionable brains are still rapidly developing.

As we learn and practice addictive eating behaviours, new electrical circuits form inside the brain that make it easier for us to continue engaging in those behaviours. As we enter adulthood, the brain undergoes a "pruning" process— dismantling circuits we don't need and keeping the circuits we use the most—so the addictive eating behaviour loops we learned in childhood become deeply etched into our minds as default pathways.

The good news is that ketogenic diets have uniquely healing properties that support the brain's ability to build brand new circuits in response to new behaviours. *So, the longer you practice your new way of eating, the stronger your healthy pathways will become. You owe it to yourself to discover what is possible.*

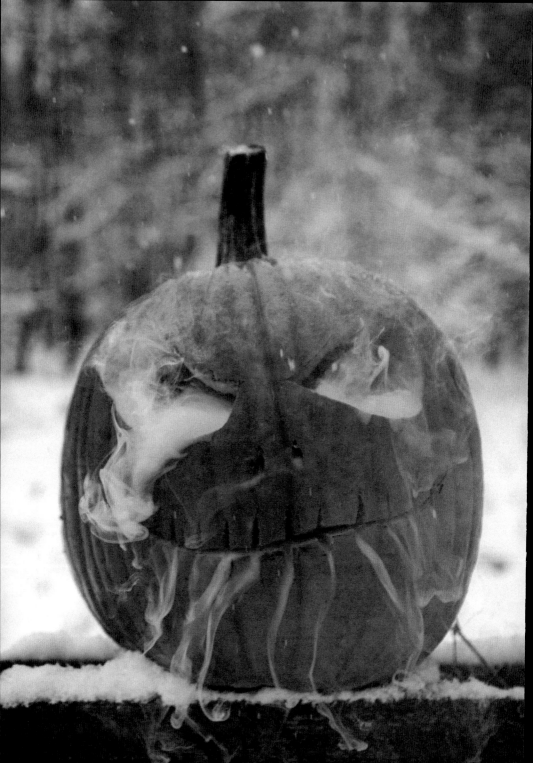

CHAPTER 6

Slips, Trips, and Falls

The cornerstone of recovery is developing and sustaining new habits of nutrition and other behaviours that help balance your brain chemistry over time

It takes time to really embed this way of living so that it feels natural and becomes who you are for life. In Chapter 5, I discussed the power of the reward system to drive you to behave in ways that you don't even want to. For this reason, carbohydrate addicts should not put their faith in willpower, however determined they are to succeed. As I said, what you have to do is simple but sometimes very hard to do.

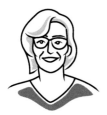

BITTEN *Every morning I tell myself: no matter what comes my way today I will stick to my food plan. Then that's taken care of for the next 24 hours, I never think about or obsess about food.*

If my Red Dog (my addicted part, craving part) comes visiting and thinks it would be a good idea to eat, for example, chocolate, I calmly tell "it" (treat it like an obnoxious 3-year-old) I hear you, but you know what, we are not doing that today. Sometimes that happens a couple of days in a row and I repeat "not today", we can all do 24 hours. Another favorite is "to tell on the Red Dog" to a friend and have a laugh about it. I have a dog, which is a big part of my recovery, I talk about dogs with friends, walk and train dogs with friends. Read about dogs. To walk alone in the woods with my dog in silence is my meditation.

I love to knit and crochet, right now dog clothes! I watch a lot of programs about space, I am a huge fan of Professor Brian Cox, sometimes I wish I was an astronomer instead of a nurse. I read a lot about neuroscience and addiction and also thrillers and literature. I spend time with my sisters living close by and nieces and nephews whenever they have time. In summer I grow roses and flowers in my tiny garden. My absolutely biggest source for recovery is nature, there is where my serenity and my solitude lie.

The primitive reward centre in our brain does its job at a very basic survival level and will always beat your logical frontal lobes.
The rational, thinking part of the brain, our consciousness, is only a small part of what is going on in our brains. We like to feel we are in control and that we have 'free will' but how often do you find this isn't the case, especially around food?

Imagine you are riding an elephant. As the rider you may be able to make it go left or right if it has been trained but so many factors other than the rider may affect the behaviour of that elephant. Is it hungry, frightened or in a bad mood? So often our conscious mind is like that rider trying to control an elephant! This helps explain why you cannot always think your way out of a craving or a relapse, your primitive brain just thunders in! Build up your new habits with determination, get to know and understand your own 'elephant'. You are heading to your dream destination, don't forget!

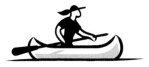

In this chapter we'll look at some of the hazards commonly encountered on your journey to food freedom and some tips on how to navigate them

Like any big journey worth undertaking there will be times when you take a wrong turn. How do you handle these setbacks and get back on track? I'll share what I have learned myself and from fellow travellers of this journey.

GEORGIA *I think it can be helpful to define what food "sobriety" means to you. For me and many of my patients, food sobriety is a feeling...a state of mind in which we are free from food preoccupation and feel in control of our food choices.*

Achieving and maintaining that peaceful, strong, resilient state of mind may require different rules for different people. For some it means keeping daily carbohydrate grams below a particular threshold, for some it means avoiding specific trigger foods, for some it means being in at least mild ketosis, for some it means weighing and measuring everything they eat.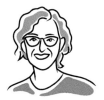

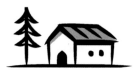 **HOME** is where you probably have most problems with addictive eating. Coming home tired from work to eat in front of the TV. Eating in the evenings and weekends. Bringing stuff back from the shops to indulge in. Cooking up your favourite carby meals and snacks. Home is where we spend most of our time.

First, remove all your trigger foods

If you can't get them all out of the house because others still want them, make sure they are out of sight. Ask family members to please indulge their chocolate habit out of your eyeline, at least for a few weeks. Make others responsible for replenishing their own stores of these foods too.

When out shopping you don't want to have the typical carb addicts' excuse of 'I'm just buying these for the kids'. Who wants to make their kids into future carb addicts anyway? Get online deliveries of food if you can and always stick to a prepared shopping list of what you need based on the delicious meals you are going to have based on protein, fat and vegetables. **Don't go shopping hungry.** Have everything ready for your evening meal or leave something in a slow cooker so that there isn't a long wait for dinner when you are hungry and tired.

WORK

Most of us spend a considerable amount of time at work. Unfortunately, most work environments have become increasingly hazardous for carb addicts. There may be biscuits and cakes in the break room or by the kettle. It seems like everyone equates carby food with treats and a good way to get through the day. It's nearly always someone's birthday, baby shower, retirement or engagement! There's probably someone who makes amazing cupcakes every Friday. If there's a canteen the food is no doubt a carbohydrate heavy disaster zone. There might even be a chocolate and crisps machine in the corridor! The work environment is full hazards.

Preparation is key

Make sure you take plenty of nutritious food that you can eat to work. I used to take breakfast and lunch. Hopefully, you have a fridge and a microwave. If not, ask if you can have them to make healthy eating easier. Bring in boxed meals. A bonus is that you will save money and can spend more on quality meat and fish. Explain to colleagues that you are trying to eat well and be ready for the carb pushers. More on that below! If you need to use the canteen choose protein with vegetables or salad.

RESTAURANTS

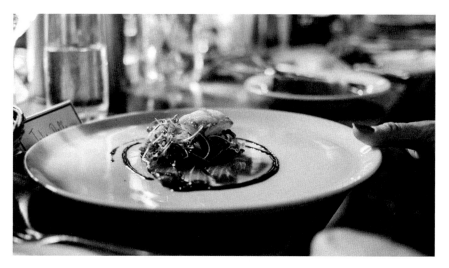

I love eating out but have learned a few lessons over the years about how to do this and still stay on track. If you are picking the restaurant it's a bit easier. You can choose somewhere that you know does meals you can eat. These days most places have their menus on line. Check it out before you go, so you can choose the best option. Usually there are starters like pate, fish or cold meats available. Most places do steak or fish dishes that you can ask for without the chips, rice or pasta they come with. Ask for extra salad or vegetables instead. If you can tolerate cheese have that as dessert or order another starter. We've never had a problem. Look out for sauces, they can sometimes have sugar in them. We ask for extra butter if we don't want the sauce. That makes anything delicious. Try not to go out super hungry so you can more easily stick to your plan.

ANNA *As long as we eat at a restaurant that serves breakfast foods or meats, I have an easy time ordering. I always ask for no seasoning, and for my meal to be prepared in bacon grease, butter or olive oil.*

DAVE *Only go if you are prepared for the challenge in front of you, have a plan on what you will be ordering. Have a list of all your food allergies to provide to the server. Do not be afraid to use the word allergy. Addiction is an allergy!*

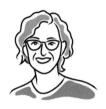

GEORGIA *If trigger foods will be present, eat something beforehand so you'll be less hungry, and plan exactly what you'll be eating when you're out. Bring something you know you can eat or choose something healthy from the menu online before leaving home and commit to ordering it. If it feels right, share your food addiction challenges with friends and family so they can support you in making good choices rather than unknowingly working against your efforts by offering you trigger foods.*

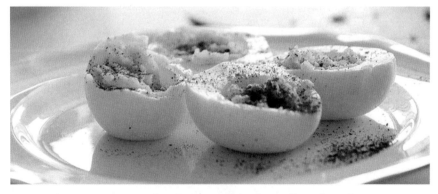

Organic eggs, avocado-oil mayo, mustard, paprika, salt and pepper

Devilled eggs are divine!

FRIENDS' HOUSES Perhaps the trickiest socially. No one wants to offend their host by not eating the food and this is probably the environment you have least control over. If they are good friends, it is a good idea to explain to them what you are doing beforehand and ask what they will be cooking.

Offer to provide some extra food of your own if you think you won't be able to eat some or part of the menu and explain that you won't be having dessert. I often ending up taking some kind of offering when I go out. I always take sparkling water too as I don't drink alcohol these days. Over the years many of our friends have joined us in our low carb journey and we now have a supper club with three other foodie couples. We each cook a course and take turns hosting.

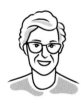

ANNA *I feel every new, interesting detail I learn about someone else, is a "treat" sweeter than anything I have ever tasted. I enjoy focusing on people, I very much like hearing about their hobbies and interests. No cake needed! I'm all in on celebrations, and refuse to feel as though I am missing out. One final tip, I usually bring something I can partake in. A platter of devilled eggs, salami and cheese, olives and dill pickles.*

BITTEN *If I am invited somewhere, I call and ask what is being served, if nothing suits me, I bring my own food. If I have guests, I cook my keto food and people love it. Nobody complains. The comment is: this food is wonderful! I felt all this was cumbersome in the beginning, I did not stand up for myself, but now it is very natural after all these years.*

BIRTHDAYS

Is it even possible to have a birthday without carbs? Well yes, it is. Just treat yourself in other ways. Buy your favourite compliant foods. For me that would be smoked salmon, maybe some scallops, filet steak. Perhaps book a night in a hotel and have the buffet breakfast (bacon, eggs, mushrooms, tomatoes). Treat yourself to a treatment or spa day. Have a day out on the train. Go to the cinema, theatre or to live music. These high days and holidays are tough at first but get easier. Make some memories.

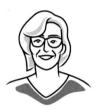

BITTEN *If I had another deadly illness and had to take medication daily (I'm grateful that I don't have to), I would not skip medication just because it is a holiday or a birthday. That's my thinking.*

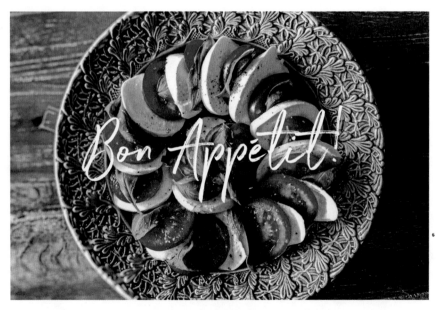

Mozzarella cheese with tomatoes, basil, olive oil, and balsamic vinegar

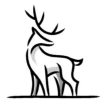

CHRISTMAS is probably the biggest single challenge to a recovering carb addict. So many triggers, expectations and extra family pressures.

I once let myself eat everything I wanted on Christmas day, telling myself it was only one day, and didn't get back into recovery until the following May. That was a very hard lesson. Each year we have refined how we do Christmas so as to make it easier and more enjoyable despite being carb free.

We stock up on good quality, seasonal food. We have wild smoked salmon and local buttered shrimps, turkey with seasoned meat stuffing, dauphinois celeriac, sprouts fried with pancetta, pigs in blankets, green beans with buttered garlic and flaked almonds, red cabbage. We buy nice cheeses with celery and walnuts along with quality coffee. We sit around a real fire, play games, listen to music and chat. David drinks Champagne, apparently it's low carb! It isn't sugar that makes occasions special, it's the company.

GEORGIA *Have fun adapting favourite holiday recipes to your food plan. We created a low-carb stuffing made entirely of ground poultry, mushrooms, celery, onions, herbs, and butter; we discovered we actually prefer it to bread stuffing, and look forward to it every year!*

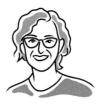

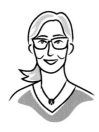

KIKI *We buy cases of sparkling water and bring bottles with us when invited for dinner and for holiday gatherings. It's our everyday beverage, but it's a special, effervescent offering at get-togethers. And a socially acceptable way for everyone to slow down on drinking alcohol and overeating food.*

HOLIDAYS

Being away from home is another difficult time for us in the beginning. I used to 'diet' before a holiday to get to a certain weight. It was a crazy mentality when I look back. I nearly always came home having put it all back on. It was as if overindulging in carbs and alcohol was the only way to have fun and relax. Now I have just as much fun and feel better for sticking to my food plan.

I don't always have breakfast now but this is very easy in hotels or if you are self-catering. Have eggs, bacon, mushrooms, tomato from the buffet. Or yoghurt, berries and seeds if they are available. Sometimes there is smoked fish. For lunch grab a big salad with chicken or fish. For dinner, steak, fish, grilled meats and vegetables or salad. Cheese if you are okay with it. If your holiday is all inclusive there will definitely be plenty of proteins and salads you can fill up on. No need at all to feel deprived or hungry.

It is easy to get plenty of activity in on holiday too; walking, swimming, cycling etc. For emergencies we often pack some almonds and vacuum-packed chorizo sausage in our luggage. David and I have travelled the world in this way and haven't had any problems so far.

GEORGIA *PCM (Phase Change Material) ice packs changed my life. Place one inside an insulated travel-friendly lunch case and your healthy perishable foods stay cold for a whole day. The packs stay solid for several hours so they pass most airport security checks!*

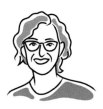

ANNA *On the road there plenty of choices available now. I can get hard boiled eggs at any convenience store, as well as many other items I occasionally eat, like cheese sticks, jerky, pork rinds, and dill pickles.*

Loved ones and other carb pushers

It may be that your family have been witness to your struggles with diet over the years and will be anxious to support you. However, it's also possible your loved ones may not understand how serious and difficult this problem is for you. As well as explaining your plan in advance, it may be helpful to ask for help so they are part of the process. After all it will help a lot if they are onboard. Also looking at it from their point of view there may be a lot less cake and 'treats' around in the future, they need to prepare. People often respond better to being asked for help rather than being given a fait accompli.

There is absolutely no doubt that you will encounter people who either genuinely believe you can't thrive without sugar and refined carbohydrate or who have their own issues with food addiction so can't be comfortable around people who have given it up. They maybe in your close family, at work or in your friendship group. It's also difficult for people who can moderate carb intake to understand that we can't. Just like people don't always understand why someone can't drink in moderation. They will tempt you and undermine you with, 'just one won't hurt', 'don't lose any more weight', 'I made it especially for you, it's your favourite', 'you look like you need some energy' or 'all that meat and fat is killing you'. They will gift you chocolates on your birthday or leave a cupcake on your desk. Sigh!

You need strategies and ready answers for these situations that you feel comfortable with. Here are some of mine:

'Oh! That's so sweet of you, it looks absolutely amazing! But I'm going to pass today because I've just eaten.'

'I love sugar — but it doesn't love me. So I'm going to have to refuse. Thank you, though'.

'It may sound crazy but if I have one piece it just makes me want more and more. So I'm much better off not having any'.

If someone persists in offering sweet or high-carb foods or bringing you them, it may be time for a bigger conversation about addiction.
Although I find most people get used to the idea after a few repetitions. I would hope that as family and friends see you feeling better, they will get on board and support you. I know it used to upset David when I was in an active addiction phase, so he was pleased to support me in my abstinence. The kids still miss the sponge puddings though! When one person changes it challenges others and you will definitely see that.

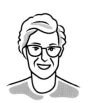 **ANNA** *Enjoy the company! Food has wrongly become an entertainment industry. Bring something you can share and enjoy or eat in advance. Be fully present in conversations. Say no gracefully. If someone doesn't know you well, just tell them you have serious allergies, and are very happy to be included in the festivities, enjoying the people and conversations. Don't be a "Debbie Downer". I love not being obsessed about food like I used to be! I enjoy socializing more now than ever before.*

Crazy cravings
Cravings can hit anytime, especially in the early days. That elephant will be lumbering around! You certainly can't think your way out of cravings very easily. Try some of these ideas:

1. **'Externalise' the craving by talking about it out loud, even if just to yourself.** 'Oh, I'm really craving X. I wonder why? Am I upset or hungry? What has triggered this craving? Etc'. 'Let's see if I can stay strong for another minute.'

2. **Have a hot or cold drink.**

3. **Take a short walk or make yourself do 10 sit ups.** Put on your favourite up beat track and do a crazy dance.

4. **If you are hungry, eat a meal based on protein and fat.**

5. **Say 'each time I resist this craving, I'm re-wiring my brain'** and have a chart on the fridge door you can tick when you resist a craving or put £1 in a tin to treat yourself to something.

6. **Message or ring someone supportive.** Maybe set this up with someone ahead of time?

7. **Make sure your home environment is trigger food free** as much as possible and avoid cook books and cooking shows on TV in the early days. Avoid social media or delete any food related groups.

ANNA *Don't put anything in your mouth that is a "drug food" for you today.*

Getting back on track

Going off course is actually part of recovery. This is how you learn what is YOUR best path. If you find yourself eating sugar and carbohydrates or other problem foods again it's time to reflect on what happened. Start with thinking about what led up to the lapse and how you would handle it differently next time? Remember, there is no failure, just the opportunity to learn from mistakes. What happened that led you off track? Were you triggered by eating or drinking just a little bit of something? Did you have too much fruit, cheese or nuts? Were you in a situation where you were too hungry and there were only bad choices to be made? Were you in a social situation and it was easier to accept the cake that turn it down? It's also time to reflect on how you feel physically and mentally having eaten trigger foods again. Sluggish, headachy, grumpy, more cravings? Make a mental note of how you would handle the situation better next time. Forgive yourself, make a plan and move on.

Get back on track as soon as you can

Do not wait for Monday morning! You are most definitely never back to square one. The pre-slip up success is still yours, you did it before and so can again. Get back on the horse quick sticks and back on your journey to food freedom. One step at a time. One day at a time. You haven't failed until you stop trying. When I look back on my own journey, I learnt some of my best lessons from what seemed at the time to be abject failure.

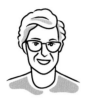

ANNA *Anyone can start over at any point during the day. Giving up is failure, relapse is an opportunity to learn perseverance, not a true failure. Successful people always fail, because they try. People who don't try can't fail, but they also can't succeed. There is no success without failure. Choose to fail forward.*

DAVE *Starting over is all about Action. Get the junk out of the house, grab a trash bag, get a supportive friend on the other end of the phone and just simply remove it.*

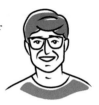

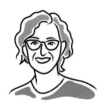

GEORGIA *I have relapsed many times. At the onset of peri-menopause, even a ketogenic diet lost its ability to control cravings and maintain my weight in a healthy range, so I experimented with a carnivore diet. A dairy-free, ketogenic, carnivore diet is the plan that seems to work best in my mid-50s to silence food preoccupation. However, it is socially, psychologically, and logistically very difficult to sustain long-term, so I strayed from it many times, and ultimately relaxed the plan to include small amounts of low-carbohydrate plant foods. When I do either unintentionally or intentionally stray from this plan, I have found fasting the next day until I am solidly in ketosis again to be a powerful recovery strategy that prevents single-day relapses from lasting many days or weeks.*

MICHAEL *I gained weight when my brother was dying after an unexpected illness and a year later when my Mom was dying with dementia. I drank more beer and wine during these stressful times. I found that doing a series of 18-, 24-, and 36-hours fasts in honor of their memory over the course of a month helped me recover physically and spiritually.*

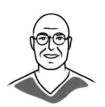

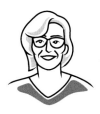

BITTEN *I relapsed several times in the beginning, there was almost no knowledge of addiction in Sweden so I tried to connect with some people in the USA and to create tools from my recovery from alcoholism. Some worked, some had to be adapted. The key to starting over, or getting back up on the horse, as I call it, is knowledge, a lot of knowledge about what relapse and recovery is, and about the addicted brain and what nourishment is needed to start rewiring the brain. And always doing an inventory of where it went wrong with my then recovery program and to always be prepared to take away things that do not work and to add new tools that will work better. Progress not perfection and to not analyse but put stuff in to action.*

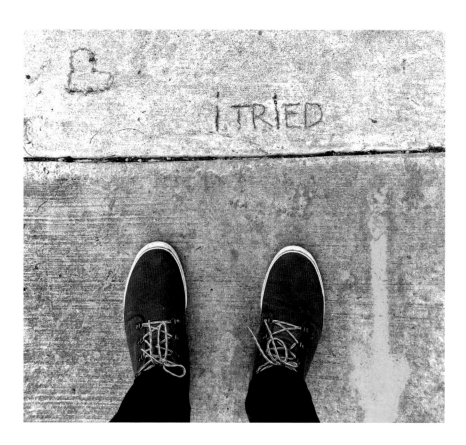

Coaches and support groups

Because we are sometimes the only food addict we know personally and because the road is long and fraught with hazards and self-sabotage and because we are social creatures, I highly recommend that you seek out some form of support for this journey. It's great to get advice and guidance from those walking the same path, especially if they are further ahead. Those people further into recovery are just like us and their success can give us hope for what we too can achieve. It's great to find others who share our experiences and be able to see that we are not alone, not to blame for our special brains and to accept the truth of our condition. There is nothing like connecting with someone else who really 'gets' it. Magic.

DAVE *I wake up, thank the universe for another day clean, hit the floor, do push ups to fatigue, read two inspirational readings. I do a recovery-based meeting from 7-8 AM. I pray before each meal and ask that the food before me serves my life and my recovery. I go through my day with gratitude and sleep well knowing I lived fully.*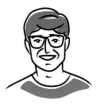

(Chapter 7 is full of information about where to go for more knowledge and support as you continue on your way.)

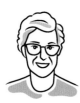 **ANNA** *Active addiction is a thief and a liar. Even as we maintain an abstinent food plan, our disease will continue to grow and change. It's a tricky, trickster. One of the biggest ways I have seen the disease trick people is by speaking to them in a little soft voice inside their head that sounds just like them and whispers "you are better now. You can relax a little. You have control. Go ahead and take one tiny little taste...it won't kill you." Listen, one bite is too many, and a thousand is never enough. The only way to recover is to stop and stay stopped.*

One way to help yourself, become more honest with yourself, is to inventory your past experiences.

Have you ever successfully eaten your trigger food for any period of time? How many times have you tried and failed to eat just one bite?

Have you rationalized and justified your eating only to find yourself in an endless loop of addictive behaviours that cause you to feel guilty and ashamed?

And finally, was it ever worth it?

Think it through, because if you are an addict like I am, you know that the temporary fix, the next high, always took you lower than the last. Why play with fire? We can learn a lot by listening to others share their experience, as well.

My friend Judy once ate one cheese curl. One cheese curl! She had been food sober for years. That one bite cost her 13 years and 80lbs. One bite!

My best advice is not to eat your trigger foods **NO MATTER WHAT.**
In fact, Judy signs every text message NMW, for no matter what. I'm not a tattoo person, but I would consider a discrete NMW somewhere!

Don't let a temporary feeling rob you of the benefits of recovery.
The freedom you have worked so hard to achieve, has given you a life free of obsession and compulsion. It's a life worth living. Once in a while, we have all had to "white knuckle it," pick up the phone and call for help, and hang on until the desire to eat something off our trigger free food plan vanishes... and it always does vanish! If I can stick to my plan until bedtime, I know you can too!

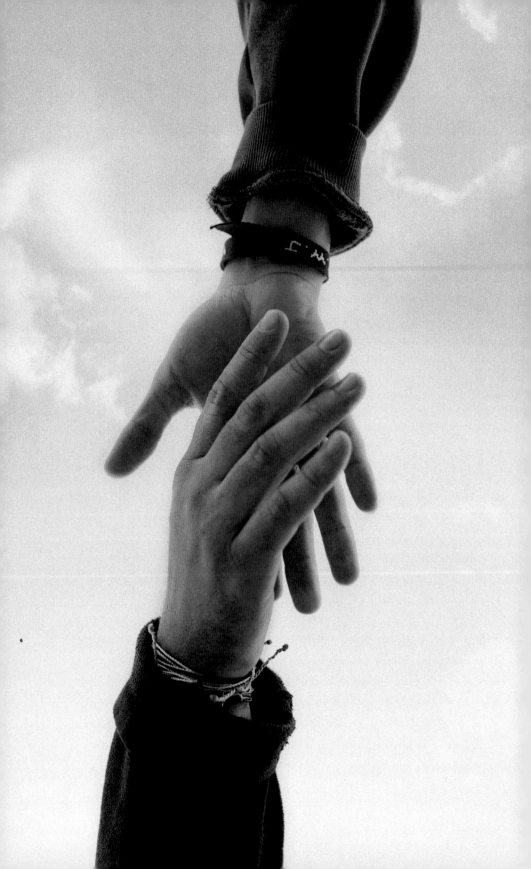

CHAPTER 7

Resources

*I'm so grateful for all the people
who have shared their knowledge and experience
with me over the last several years
of my journey.*

*Here are people, books, websites and apps I have found most helpful.
The list isn't exhaustive, of course, but I hope you will find other resources
and people who help you on your way. I'll be blogging and updating
resources and recipes on my website.*

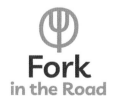

ForkInTheRoad.co.uk

FOOD ADDICTION

ForkInTheRoad.co.uk
My website and where I feature interviews with recovering food addicts, blog updates and resources as I find them.

BittensAddiction.com
Bitten Jonsson is one of the best-known clinicians in sugar addiction. She trains professionals to assess and treat the condition. Her Facebook group, *Sugarbomb In Your Brain,* is an excellent source of support and good information.

SUGARxGlobal.com
Set up by Anna, Dave, and other amazing sugar addiction counsellors in the USA with lots of useful information about how to recover and find support.

DrJoanIfland.com
Joan Ifland has written the definitive text book on processed food addiction. She runs an online support community.

RobertLustig.com
Dr Robert Lustig is internationally known for his work on the damage sugar does to our bodies and minds, fostering today's epidemics of addiction and depression.

AddictionsUnplugged.com
Dr Vera Tarman is a carb addiction expert and is the author of *Food Junkies.*

BOOKS

The Yoga of Eating
Charles Eisenstein

2003

The Sugar Demons
Johnathan Cranford

2020

Fat Chance
Dr Robert Lustig

2014

In the Realm of the Hungry Ghosts
Gabor Mate

2018

Food Junkies
Vera Tarman

2014

Processed Food Addiction
Joan Ifland et al. 2018.

Unfit for Purpose
Adam Hart

2020

Escape the Diet Trap
Dr John Briffa

2012

Nutrition and Recipes

DietDoctor.com

Probably the world's biggest website devoted to the benefits of low carb and ketogenic diets. A mine of information. Remember that carb addicts should avoid sweeteners and alcohol even if they are allowed on other plans.

Diabetes.co.uk

The world's largest on-line community for people with diabetes and supports people via online forums and also runs the www.lowcarbprogram.com on line subscription program with weekly support, recipes and tips for going low carb.

PaleoCanteen.co.uk

Producers of paleo and low carb food in the UK.
Visit their blog and recipe book, too.

PHCuk.org

The PHC is a UK charity campaigning to improve public health by providing quality information. Author profits from this book will be donated to the Public Health Collaboration. You can find Dr Unwin's sugar infographics at PHCuk.org/sugar as well as up to date summaries of the latest low carb research.

LowCarbTogether.com

Is a beautiful website designed to help you on your low carb journey. It's hosted by my favourite foodies Katie and Giancarlo Caldesi. Katie's low carb recipe books are stunning and are available on the website or Amazon.
Katie also has a Facebook group.

Recovery Resources

This great podcast by Dr Vera Varman, Molly Painschab and
Clarissa Kennedy is wonderful. They are all so knowledgeable as practitioners
in the field as well as having their own carb addiction stories.
They interview researchers and practitioners in the field.
FoodJunkies.libsyn.com

A great website with a recovery podcast
UnsweetenedSio.com

Practice Meditation and Mindfulness
Both have apps for your phone.
Calm.com
Headspace.com

Learn Yoga
For yoga, try and find a local class or do an online class to get started.
YogaWithAdriene.com

Find a New Hobby
Hobbies help. Volunteering for a local good cause
is another idea to boost your wellbeing.
HobbyHelp.com
HobbyLark.com

Discover Your Character Strengths
A free test is available at Prof Martin Seligman's website
AuthenticHappiness.sas.upenn.edu
Under Questionnaires » A Brief Strengths Test

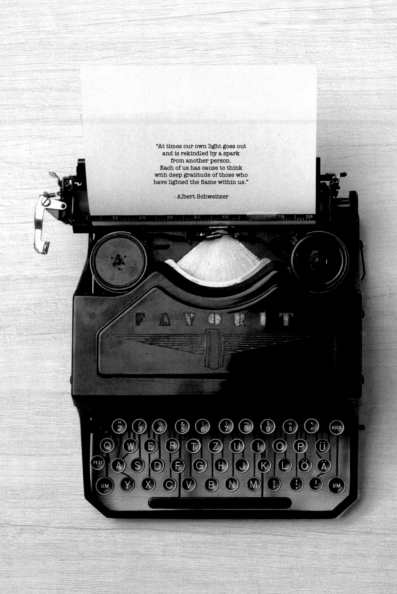

"At times our own light goes out
and is rekindled by a spark
from another person.
Each of us has cause to think
with deep gratitude of those who
have lighted the flame within us."

- Albert Schweitzer

Acknowledgments

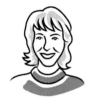
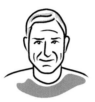
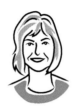
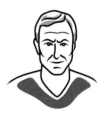

HEIDI GIAEVER @VerHeidi

DAVID HOYLE @THPcoaching

ELOISE NEELEY @EloiseNeeley

DR GARY TAUBES @GaryTaubes

With grateful thanks

*To our friends and colleagues who kindly commented
on early drafts and shared their time and wisdom*

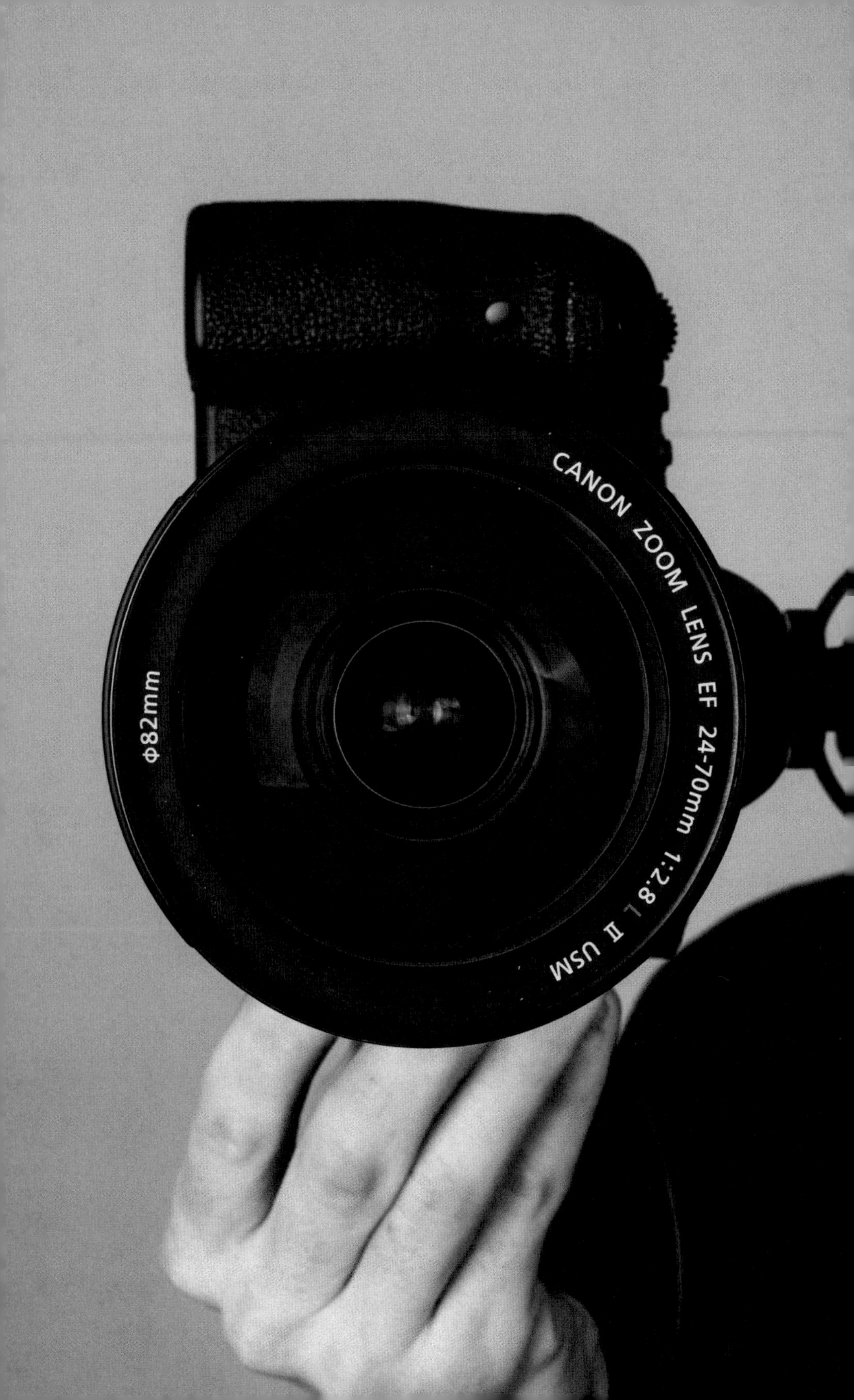
CANON ZOOM LENS EF 24-70mm 1:2.8 L II USM
Φ82mm

Thanks to Our Featured Artists

Thank You!

PHC is a charity dedicated to informing and implementing healthy decisions for better public health. We publish evidence-based reports on the most pressing public health issues alongside coordinated campaigns and implementing initiatives for improving public health.

*Our funding comes from profits from books,
newsletter subscriptions, the sale of t-shirts, and from
individual donations and memberships by fantastic people like you.
You can quick-donate £2 by SMS texting "PHC" to 70660*

Public Health Collaboration
Visit us at PHCuk.org

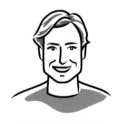

SAM FELTHAM
 @PHCukorg

Charity No. 1171887